MW01167182

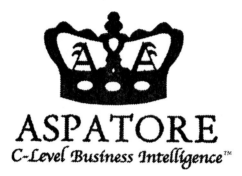

ASPATORE
C-Level Business Intelligence™

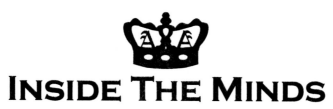

INSIDE THE MINDS

Empowering Professionals of All Levels
With C-Level Business Intelligence
www.InsideTheMinds.com

The critically acclaimed *Inside the Minds* series provides readers of all levels with proven business intelligence from C-Level executives (CEO, CFO, CTO, CMO, Partner) from the world's most respected companies. Each chapter is comparable to a white paper or essay and is a future-oriented look at where an industry/profession/topic is heading and the most important issues for future success. Each author has been carefully chosen through an exhaustive selection process by the *Inside the Minds* editorial board to write a chapter for this book. *Inside the Minds* was conceived in order to give readers actual insights into the leading minds of business executives worldwide. Because so few books or other publications are actually written by executives in industry, *Inside the Minds* presents an unprecedented look at various industries and professions never before available. The *Inside the Minds* series is revolutionizing the business book market by To nominate yourself, another individual, or a group of executives for an upcoming Inside the Minds book, or to suggest a specific topic for an Inside the Minds book, please email jason@aspatore.com.

For information on bulk orders, sponsorship opportunities or any other questions, please email store@aspatore.com.

For information on licensing the content in this book, or any content published by Aspatore, please email jennifer@aspatore.com.

To nominate yourself, another individual, or a group of executives for an upcoming Inside the Minds book, or to suggest a specific topic for an Inside the Minds book, please email jason@aspatore.com.

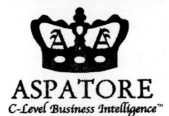

ASPATORE
C-Level Business Intelligence™

www.Aspatore.com

Aspatore publishes only the biggest names in the business world, including C-Level leaders (CEO, CTO, CFO, COO, CMO, Partner) from over half the world's 500 largest companies and other leading professionals (such as doctors and lawyers). By focusing on publishing only C-Level executives, Aspatore provides professionals of all levels with proven business intelligence from industry insiders, rather than relying on the knowledge of unknown authors and analysts. Aspatore publishes a highly innovative line of business intelligence publications including Inside the Minds, Bigwig Briefs, ExecRecs, Business Travel Bible, Brainstormers, The C-Level Test, and Aspatore Business Reviews, in addition to other best selling business books, journals and briefs. Aspatore focuses on publishing traditional print books with individuals, while our portfolio companies, Corporate Publishing Group (B2B Writing & Editing) and ExecEnablers (business intelligence stores) focus on developing areas within the business and publishing worlds.

CORPORATE PUBLISHING GROUP
Outsource Your Company's
Writing & Editing To the World's Best

www.CorporatePublishingGroup.com

Corporate Publishing Group (CPG) provides companies with on-demand writing and editing resources from the world's best writing teams. Our clients come to CPG for the writing and editing of books, reports, speeches, company brochures, press releases, product literature, web site copy and other publications. This enables companies to save time and money, reduce headcount, and ensure polished and articulate written pieces. Each client is assigned a CPG team devoted to their company, which works on their projects throughout the course of a year on an as-needed basis and helps generate new written documents, review and edit documents already written, and provide an outside perspective before a document "goes public" in order to help companies maintain a polished image both internally and externally. All projects outsourced to CPG are developed according to the strict specifications of the client, and delivered on a specific deadline. Clients have included companies in all industries and disciplines, ranging from financial to technology to law firms, and are represented by over half of the Fortune 500. For more information please e-mail jonp@corporatepublishinggroup.com or visit our web site at www.CorporatePublishingGroup.com.

INSIDE THE MINDS:
The Art & Science of
Being a Doctor

*Leading Doctors Reveal the Secrets to Professional
and Personal Success as a Doctor*

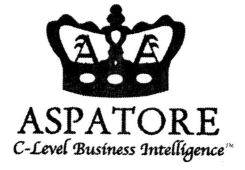

ASPATORE
C-Level Business Intelligence™

If you are interested in purchasing bulk copies for your team/company with your company logo, or for sponsorship, promotions or advertising opportunities, please email store@aspatore.com or call toll free 1-866-Aspatore.

Published by Aspatore Books, Inc.
For corrections, company/title updates, comments or any other inquiries please email info@aspatore.com.

First Printing, 2002
10 9 8 7 6 5 4 3 2 1

ISBN 1-58762-119-3

Edited by Jo Alice Hughes, Proofread by Ginger Conlon, Cover design by Kara Yates & Ian Mazie

Material in this book is for educational purposes only. This book is sold with the understanding that neither any of the authors or the publisher is engaged in rendering medical, legal, accounting, investment, or any other professional service. For medical help, please contact your doctor.

This book is printed on acid free paper.

A special thanks to all the individuals that made this book possible.

Special thanks to: Kirsten Catanzano, Melissa Conradi, Molly Logan, Justin Hallberg

The views expressed by the individuals in this book do not necessarily reflect the views shared by the companies they are employed by (or the companies mentioned in this book). The companies referenced may not be the same company that the individual works for since the publishing of this book.

INSIDE THE MINDS:
The Art & Science of Being a Doctor

CONTENTS

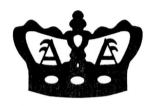

PRACTICING TO A HIGHER STANDARD: PATIENT FIRST

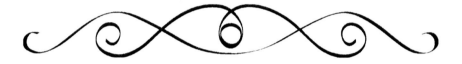

W. RANDOLPH CHITWOOD, JR., M.D.
East Carolina University
Brody School of Medicine

Department of Surgery
Professor and Chairman

The Art, the Science, and the Physician's Path

The essence of medicine can best be understood by considering it a true profession, encompassing both art and science. It is this unity and the unique application of these disciplines that make a good physician. Adding unswerving commitment and ethical behavior makes a great doctor. The intertwining of these qualities makes medicine a challenge with many rewards, but also many demands. This profession, more than any other, affects both the physical nature and the emotional behavior of not only the patient, but also the family. This alone is why the three learned professions were considered to be medicine, law, and the clergy. They all affect the true being of a person – how one feels about oneself. A special, continuing trust and bonding relationship can evolve from a positive physician encounter during stressful times, and this bond is usually amplified and preserved, especially when a patient's health is restored. The art and science of medicine have been inextricably interrelated for centuries, albeit with less advanced technology than today.

The *art of medicine,* first practiced by Galen and the early Greek physicians, preceded by centuries the science and technology of medicine as they are known today. On a superficial level, without a true understanding of the significance of doctor-patient communications, some might think the art is simply a good bedside manner. The ability to listen to patients, recognize and understand their needs, and show compassionate feelings for them and their families has a therapeutic benefit for the patient. Such encounters often relieve much of the anxiety of families, while giving the physician the opportunity to truly observe his or her patients in a more comfortable, natural milieu. The complexity of biological systems, as well as the interdependence of the mind and body, demands that the profession incorporate every aspect of the patient in the care provided.

Physicians practicing the art of medicine optimally develop a sixth sense – an uncanny ability to use deductive reasoning, often without having much hard data – in approaching the patient's illness. This sixth sense generally evolves to an instinctive skill, which allows the doctor to piece together a myriad of symptoms and laboratory results to complete the diagnostic puzzle. This important ingredient develops only with experience, observation, scientific knowledge, and dedication to medicine. Doctors of the past often relied on this innate understanding more than on diagnostic testing. Unfortunately, many physicians today have reversed this trend and rely less on complete understanding of a patient's history, physical findings, and emotional complement.

The *science of medicine* is distinct from the art of medicine, although each is dependent on the other. The doctor who understands the art of medicine generally understands the science, which in turn perpetually enhances the art of the profession. The science of medicine requires a database of knowledge acquired over years through reading, research, observation, and experience. The basis of medical scientific education, both clinical and natural science, is initially obtained in college and medical school. The more formal curriculum concludes with a residency program and may last up to 10 years following medical school. During this period doctors learn to apply what they have learned and make constant improvements by an iterative process and observation of their results. Appropriate senior supervision guides the resident's hand toward the right decisions for patient care. This period does not preserve the classical "walls" present in most educations, but subtends a broader environment of the clinics and hospital wards.

Following this closely mentored training and study, the doctor is ready to begin a new learning experience in his or her practice. This is a special time, as it signifies the beginning of a more introspective personal education for the young doctor. It is a time during which many of us learn as much about ourselves as we learn about our patients.

One of the first obligations of physicians, both young and mature, is to keep abreast of new scientific information. The complexity and speed with which knowledge is generated and communicated today make it imperative to stay current, not only on the advances in global medicine and one's specialty, but with regard to the general advances made in science and technology. Each of these may relate indirectly to medicine and new medical developments. Today Internet communication and rapid worldwide data transfer have enhanced our ability to keep up-to-date scientifically.

Surgical specialties also demand the development of adroit physical abilities that include fine spatial manual dexterity, often embracing ambidexterity. Moreover, these talents must be linked to an in-depth understanding of anatomy and physiology. Many of these skills can be acquired through practice and observation, while others remain individual and innate. Daily, surgeons apply base knowledge through manual dexterity to effect a cure for their patients, often without the benefit of a long analysis. The distinction between cognitive skills and technical applications here becomes blurred in most situations, as they are interlinked.

Combining the Art and Science to Benefit the Patient

The individual seeking and accepting the role of physician takes on a unique responsibility to each patient, as well as to the public. The lifestyle of a good doctor should remain apart from the herd. As physicians are observed more often and more closely than others, they should remain responsible at all times. Being a doctor becomes part of a person's being with an almost continuous consciousness of this responsibility. The expectation of the community generally is that physicians should be held in high esteem and respected. However, the character of the person who is called "Doctor" defines this realization. These responsibilities and expectations should influence all of the physician's interactions within the profession and community. Daily foibles, such as unbridled anger, lack of verbal etiquette, and loss of control can impair an otherwise superb physician and rob him or her of public respect. The stresses of the day have impaired many excellent doctors through substance abuse, emotional instability, and lack of control. The preeminent physician Sir William Osler (1849-1919) once said physicians must "educate your nerve centers" and act with imperturbability — displaying "coolness and presence of mind under all circumstances." He considered this latter quality that most

[handwritten marginalia: yeah; oh?; you must appear perfect?; a real identity; I know someone who can do that, par excellence]

appreciated by the laity. These maxims hold as true today as they did on the day he wrote them early in the last century.

One of the most essential qualities in a doctor is honesty, which includes all professional practice, with colleagues, in the hospital, with patients, and in personal life. Most important, the doctor must maintain self-honesty, which allows one to assess personal actions and review medical outcomes. The true doctor is one who can be introspective personally and professionally.

I believe doctors have the obligation to conduct themselves according to high moral standards, much as Boy Scouts are to follow a moral code of behavior. It is important for doctors to set ethical standards for themselves, for both their personal life and their medical practice. Accepting the responsibility for patients' illnesses, and in many cases their lives, requires the physician to live by a high ethical standard; this is essential for the best treatment and care of the patient.

The physician needs to be an intelligent person with an almost insatiable desire to keep learning. Driven by intellectual curiosity and the need to satisfy self-imposed standards of medical learning and practice, doctors should pursue knowledge, even in time spent on non-medical matters. They must enjoy the pursuit of lifelong learning. This continuous learning allows the best application of the right treatment and best medical care within the scope of resources available to the patient. The term "holistic" has become a cliché for an understanding of the patient as a whole person with the inseparable workings of the mind and body. Treating patients thus requires the doctor to be a person

all this stuff is, oddly enough, kind of de-humanizing. It certainly keeps a Dr. out of touch.

who understands this concept and brings it to the bedside. Patients are affected by many things – not only their physical ailments – and the best doctors truly hear what patients are saying and fully understand the impact of emotions on illness, as well as prospective treatments and outcomes.

Communication skills are quintessential for the effective doctor. Patients and families must have the best possible understanding of the illness, treatment options, and prognosis. Again, hearing what patients and family members are saying not only enhances the patient's understanding, but engenders more comfort and confidence in the doctor entrusted with the care. Communicating with patients consists of more than just advice; the doctor's words may be the patient's only solace, especially when no treatment is available or appropriate. The physician needs to communicate with family members. Beyond their personal need for understanding, they are the ones who will become extended caregivers. Osler, an early 20th century ethicist at Johns Hopkins, said, "It is much more important to know what sort of patient has the disease than what sort of disease the patient has." The doctor needs good communication skills to bring the art and science of medicine together for the benefit of the patient.

Keeping up-to-date and practicing medicine, with its constant advances, as well as being a compassionate communicator, would seem to be enough for any professional person. However, the demands on the physician extend much further. Physicians set standards for themselves and also follow practice guidelines. It is these personal standards that should demand the most from the physician. Physicians should become involved in hospital medical staff activities and communicate effectively with the hospital administration. Who other than these frontline caregivers can better determine the adequacy of the facility or quality of medical practice in the hospital? It is at the administrative and board of trustee levels that decisions are made on the purchasing of medical equipment and staff appointments. Quality assurance has become synonymous with always being sure the best possible care is provided and that monitoring mechanisms are effective. Only involved physicians can know and influence these activities to create the best hospital practices. Active hospital participation should include support for in-house continuing education of peers and staff, as well as the community. Patients frequently tell their doctors of their experiences at the hospital, good and bad. Both concerns and compliments must be passed on to the administrative decision-makers. The physician needs to be concerned about the professional activity of the other hospital caregivers and how they are treating patients. The doctor must always be the patient's advocate, both for safety and for support, during the stressful time of a hospital stay.

There is one additional arena that cannot be ignored: the health of the people in the community – public health. Many of the illnesses requiring treatment start years before we first see patients present with symptoms. Many of their illnesses are preventable or can be controlled. Education and early detection are essential components of public health. Physicians who support community public health, practice preventive medicine in their offices, and make their voices heard in community forums supplement their effectiveness.

and private practice!

Prevailing through medical school, internship, and residency requires long hours and hard work. It is the tenacity to see an undertaking to completion that initially distinguishes young doctors and gains the respect of others. However, *what is that?* notwithstanding this respect, the doctor must maintain this pace and commitment. The penchant for hard work must be an essential characteristic of the practicing physician. Today lifestyle alterations are becoming more important than the professional life for many doctors. Also, the unbridled pursuit of economic goals by practitioners can disconnect them from the respect they have worked so hard to earn. When either of these latter issues becomes the primary nucleus of a doctor's life, then it is appropriate for the public to remove this doctor from the list of those regarded as "professional."

the "sleazy" surgeon

The Personal-Professional Balance

Many of us find it impossible to disconnect from patient responsibilities at the end of the day or workweek. It is difficult to gain respite from all responsibilities; however, periodic vacations are a must for the sake of personal health and family happiness. Achieving a balance between personal and professional life requires each doctor to do what is right for himself or herself. I find this balance easily, as I have many hobbies that meld very nicely with my professional life. Each hobby has a synergistic effect on the other and forms a continuum with my work. Two examples of how hobbies and medicine work together for me are my serious interest in photography and my past interest in ham radio.

HA I know the kids a bone

My knowledge of radio communications has given me an appreciation and understanding of technology that translates to an understanding of many of the newer types of equipment we use in the hospital, such as those controlled by computers. My experience with photography has been extremely useful in diagnostic imaging and in the use of the three-dimensional screen of the Da Vinci® robot in the operating room.

Balance between personal and professional life will be achieved when the doctor can feel that the system he or she works in is delivering the care he or she wants to deliver to patients. When a doctor is dissatisfied with the work environment, it may not be possible to maintain a balance in life.

I wonder if that's what happened w/ SEGO

In addition, I believe that achieving satisfaction in life requires the doctor to have some protected time or personal time to enjoy the pleasures of family or to pursue the hobbies that offer the opportunity to relax and recover energy spent in the practice of medicine. This balance will afford the doctor the time to keep fresh within the profession and to satisfy natural curiosities.

The Physician and Goal-setting

Success in any profession depends on planning, whether one is in the training period to enter a profession or is already a functioning professional. Primary to any planning, I believe, is the setting of a goal. Having a goal sets a pathway to one's objective and facilitates the development of strategies to meet that goal.

what if you don't know how to plan?

I've only ever set personal goals

18

As a physician with serious concern for patients and their illnesses, I find goals can take the form of developing the ultimate treatment or setting a clinical pathway for treatment. The development of new technologies or the refinement of present equipment can also be valuable goals. The best way to pursue goals of this nature, or those relating to a daily practice, is through continuing education by the doctor. Going forward or being on the cutting edge in the practice of medicine requires the doctor to be current on all medical research and new technologies.

Goals will need to be reset as they are reached or as experience dictates. It is important to remember that achieving goals will frequently depend on allowing other individuals or an institution to give their support to the endeavor.

My strategy for setting goals includes establishing a timeline for the execution of the various phases of the plan. The financial portion of the plan must have a detailed listing of resources needed and resources available. In addition, planning for other sources of financial support is critical.

Planning must also consider obstructions that could arise, along with legal or regulatory obstacles that exist or may develop. Ethical issues must be considered from the point of view of personal values and from the point of view of the institution, the practice of medicine, and the patient. *That pesky ole patient! Just like all that damn singin' at the opera!!*

All physicians need to develop planning and evaluation techniques to function smoothly in their practices and to experience the success of their work. Goal-setting is an ongoing process that can allow the doctor to take alternate pathways in the treatment of disease and in reaching personal goals.

Not infrequently, setting goals to achieve high levels of patient care or development of some innovative equipment or treatment can lead to frustration. However, in many cases the physician trained in goal-setting and planning will turn the frustration into a drive to do something new for the patient and for medicine.

The Challenging Aspects of Being a Doctor

I find medicine a continuous challenge, including all aspects of practice. The advances made every day in medicine make it imperative that physicians keep abreast of new developments. More new information has arisen in the past 10 years than in the past 100 years. The ever-increasing patient disease and psychosocial complexities increase this challenge. Rarely do we see patients with a single disease entity or uncomplicated social situation. Moreover, the aging population has placed both volume and complexity demands on physicians, as well as on the ever-changing healthcare delivery system. Guidelines, assessments, and limitations are imposed increasingly on the practice of medicine that do not seem to be linked to patient care. Moreover, the economic situation in healthcare has become more limiting and in the future may preclude access to healthcare for many people. Clearly, many of these converging problems will challenge our young doctors and their successors even more.

Perhaps one of the greatest challenges for the physician is working with other physicians in a team approach to affect the best patient outcomes. Working together will ensure maximal combined expertise and minimize any potential for error. The patient benefits most from a cohesive, coordinated effort, and each physician can benefit from added insight, knowledge, and collegiality. Working together will reinforce future efforts and improve patient care. Unfortunately, today economic alliances can preclude the best doctors in the community from coming together as a cohesive force. This is regrettable for both the patient and physician professionalism. I believe this cohesiveness must be reestablished. Fortunately, in areas of less competition and incomplete managed care penetration, cohesive relations exist among individual groups and solo practitioners.

As mentioned, the aging population is challenging modern medical practice more than ever. This group brings complex, chronic diseases along with demands for the latest in medical treatments. In addition, many present combinations of co-morbidities, making treatment difficult at best. Treating each illness, while avoiding conflicts between treatments and drugs and meeting the demands of a population seeking an active and productive life, is a challenge for every doctor today. It is interesting that in the past physicians had less to offer in terms of therapy, and to a healthier population, but more time to spend with each patient. Oddly, this ratio has reversed because of the increasing number of complex patients.

For example, the aging population experiences frequent medication complications, often because of their inability to follow treatment recommendations. For those with later, even subtle, mental changes, the challenges also include safety and caregiver concerns. An elderly caregiver may become the person needing the greatest attention. Although the science of medicine in making a diagnosis and prescribing the best treatment may be foremost in the physician's mind, the art of working with patients of all ages and their families is a great challenge and is becoming an even greater one. Often elderly patients want to live independently, but when they become debilitated, the family response is neglect because of work arrangements, lack of family cohesion, inadequate means, or any combination thereof. The physician often becomes the intermediary, brokering care through extended living arrangements, more frequent doctor visits, or family counseling. This is a role that many physicians had little involvement in 25 years ago, as family structures were different, and "elderly patients" were a younger set than those seen today.

AH HA!

The doctor's efforts to save lives and alleviate patient suffering are not always successful. As an experienced cardiac surgeon I often operate on very ill patients, some with few options. Many of these patients are elderly, with multiple medical conditions that make them high-risk. In many instances, it is appropriate to perform a complex heart operation despite the risks. Even knowing these risks does not help the family or the surgeon become conditioned when the patient does not survive. Even more perplexing are circumstances that are worse than mortality. For example, the surgeon may get the patient through surgery, but when a stroke or respiratory insufficiency occurs, the patient is not restored to the lifestyle he or she had hoped for. Clearly, this is one of the most difficult aspects of being a surgeon. The same things occur in any physician's mind when the results obtained are less than optimal. This is a part of medicine, but the best doctors never become accustomed to or really accept failure. Our credo is to restore health to our patients and to do no harm – this is the essence of our profession. *It's not about the patient – it's about the doctor.*

When apparently at a roadblock in treating one of my patients, I *frequently*. *That was where* consider the alternative pathways available. As the patient's *hanis* advocate, I take seriously my responsibility in finding a *folder* treatment that affords the patient an opportunity for a cure or *excelled* amelioration of his or her illness or pain, whatever is the best *it was* that can be achieved, considering the situation. *about the patient.*

Great resources are available to me in seeking an alternative treatment if my first choice is not suitable for some reason. Consulting with other physicians and specialists in the area is always available to the doctor. Bringing others' knowledge and experience to the situation may uncover some approach to the problem that is satisfactory for my patient. Additionally, I have medical literature available to search for an alternate methodology that has been tried and tested by other physicians.

In other situations, searching for new ways to get patients to treatment may not be centered on the illness, but on the payment of the treatment and the hospital's use and care. Here again, I seek alternative funding so my patient can receive the needed care.

Constant Change: Challenges and Satisfaction

Physicians practicing over the past several decades have seen marked changes in the healthcare system and in the care of the hospitalized patient. The passage of Medicare and Medicaid legislation in the early 1960s first provided greater access to care for the patients and better reimbursement for the physicians. However, within the past 10 years these funds have retrenched to the point that care has become threatened, and access to care will surely decline for our elderly and less wealthy patients. Not only have these funds decreased for physician payment, but hospital reimbursement has also fallen drastically.

These factors effect not only patient care, but also medical student, postgraduate, and specialty training. Moreover, funds for basic and clinical research are severely threatened and dwindling. The academic medical center, once the cornerstone of innovation and discovery, as well as physician education, is now threatened more than ever, and many of these institutions are near closure. The American public expects the best medical care. This includes new technology, new discoveries, and well-trained physicians. No doubt in the near future a complete reassessment of federal, state, private insurance, and managed-care funding will need to be addressed in the face of decreasing care quality and access. While physicians must keep abreast of all new scientific findings, their judgment in the choice of treatment and clinical activity may be altered by government regulations. Physicians have lost a great deal of autonomy in treating their patients.

For example, the federal government's demand for shorter hospital stays has influenced, and in some situations determined, the actions of the doctor who must comply with all regulations. The hospital often pressures the doctor to discharge patients as soon as possible. Limits set by private healthcare insurers also put restrictions on the doctor and the hospital. Clearly, we must be concerned about the cost of healthcare; however, at the same time we must continue to advocate the best treatments for our patients.

Although the requirements imposed by insurance companies present a challenge, the uninsured also pose a financial problem for both the doctor and healthcare institutions. Finances are squeezed from other angles, as well. For example, the filing of lawsuits by patients and their families puts pressure and expense on the physician, who must have ample malpractice insurance. Frequent lawsuits, many without merit, have compelled some insurers to cancel or totally withdraw from providing malpractice insurance. This creates another difficulty for the practicing physician.

But in spite of all of these difficulties, many medical advances have added to the excitement of practicing medicine. Great advances in the discovery of drugs and their increased effectiveness in the treatment of some formerly untreatable diseases afford the doctor the satisfaction of success in patient care.

The advances in diagnostic tools have been exciting for the doctor and have simplified many procedures once thought necessary for an accurate diagnosis. Patients have benefited greatly from newer imaging technology, avoiding the more invasive aspects of exploratory surgical procedures for diagnosis.

These advances have led to less invasive techniques for treating illnesses. Endoscopic techniques in the operating room have resulted in fewer traumas to the patient needing surgery, less discomfort for the patient, and shortened hospital stays. Although the advances in technology already allow surgeons to perform surgery with fewer traumas to the patient, the future holds promise of even greater advances in this area.

In the future, medicine will be driven even more by technology. The operating room is in a revolution of advances, as evidenced by robotic surgery, the ultimate in less invasive surgery. It is practiced in many locations around the world. Medical school settings are preparing the best of surgeons to perform surgery with this advanced equipment.

Nanotechnology, making equipment smaller, will be another advance in medical practice that will contribute to smaller implants and smaller equipment used in less invasive techniques.

Telemedicine will also benefit the home healthcare patient by adding visual images to the communications between the doctor and the caregivers in the home setting. Telemedicine will also increase the ability of practitioner-teachers to share patient experiences with other physicians without having to leave home base.

Research findings relating to the genome – along with the application of these findings in understanding the basis of disease, the treatment of disease, and hopefully its prevention – can only challenge the scientific minds of physicians and their desire to bring the latest to their patients. This increased knowledge will bring the doctor to a better understanding of the true basis of disease.

Increasing medical records' use of the computer will provide the physician with easy access to all patient data, assisting in and ensuring a more accurate diagnosis and comprehensive care. The computer and Internet give the physician and the public access to medical information, and as this area matures, it will provide a stronger database of current research and up-to-date medical thinking for the doctor.

Members of the general public already use the Internet to search for an understanding of their illnesses, and this research will make them more active participants in their own care, which can enhance the communications between doctor and patient.

These advances in technology and information, I believe, will contribute to the emergence of the specialist in medical practice, such as the cardiovascular surgeon. The generalist will be the entry level of medicine.

I believe, as do others, that the future will see a continuation in the speed of change in medicine, and that the changes will be both a challenge and a source of satisfaction for us all. The advances promise much to both the ill person and the practicing physician.

When asked what I would do if I could create any new drug in the world or cure any disease, I would respond without hesitation: I would like to create a new drug that would cure viral illnesses. Through the use of this drug many infectious diseases and many malignancies could be cured or stopped. Such a drug could have a tremendous impact on the world's health and social well-being. An endeavor of such magnitude would require the development of an initiative, collaboration with pharmaceutical companies and the National Institutes of Health, and the involvement of many different scientists with various types of expertise.

Doctors as Leaders

Personal success begins early, when a doctor receives a good basic training in medicine, which is then continuously fed by his or her intellectual curiosity. This curiosity is a force that will need the continuous nourishment of current scientific and updated medical information.

To satisfy their curious minds, doctors must read the scientific and medical literature. In addition, attendance at medical conferences exposes doctors to the latest information and enables the exchange of ideas between active minds. These activities will add to the continuous growth of the doctors in the profession and prepare them to teach courses for colleagues and the support staff at the hospital. Teaching courses will enable physicians to synthesize their experiences and knowledge into a comprehensive understanding, gain opportunities to contribute to the profession, and increase leadership skills. These activities will prepare doctors for certification and recertification in medical specialties.

If the profession is to move forward in technology and the giving of care, it is essential for all doctors to continue learning and sharing knowledge. I find that personal studies, teaching, and writing will add to a physician's growth, as will learning from other physicians' skills and behaviors.

Pursuing an understanding of technology and its advances, especially as they are applied to medical practice, is fundamental for physicians if they are to be used to their fullest advantage. I see the physician as not only understanding and using technology, but also applying the knowledge gained to meet the needs of the future. Innovations in technology by the physician will enhance medical practice for the benefit of patients.

An example of such an innovation I am presently working with and training surgeons to apply to their patients is robotic surgery. This less invasive advance in surgery will benefit the patient by reducing the trauma and discomfort of surgery and shortening the hospital stay. Bringing technology to the future and even creating the future of medicine is a measure of personal and professional success.

The physician also has a role as a team member or team leader within the clinical area. Initially it is essential that the doctor know the objectives of the group's efforts and share the same goals with the other team members. Dedication and commitment to meeting those goals require good communication skills with all team members, and most important, a high ethical and moral approach to the problem at hand.

Team membership may require that the physician develop some increased technical skills when appropriate to help meet the team's objective. Included among these skills may be surgical, data coordination, profusion, and robotic surgery skills.

While working with other doctors, I observe and respect the many skills they bring to medicine. It is their ability to treat patients effectively, sometimes with limited resources, that reminds me that most physicians are in the profession for the right reasons. Although we are all faced with the changing times and perhaps negative influences on the conscientious practice of medicine, many continue to preserve their personal and professional standards. The physician who has that extra caring will study the ethical issues facing medicine today and incorporate this thinking into his or her daily practice.

Being a good clinician is the basic quality of a leader in medicine. Early in my medical career, I learned that hard work is essential to be a good clinician. I soon realized that it is part of every aspect of being a doctor, especially a leader in the profession. Working as a physician got me involved with many local issues and activities, and I see this as inevitable for the doctor working within the community.

Another quality I see as necessary in a leader is the ability to think globally about issues that extend beyond the field of medicine. Tenacity to see a problem through to some conclusion is a characteristic I'd expect to see in a leader in medicine. Imperturbability in working with others in the profession is necessary for smooth working relationships within the clinical area, as is the ability to work with a group and be able to foster a single group opinion. An important quality for personal and professional growth is the ability to take criticism and learn from mistakes.

Leadership in medicine can take many forms. Some doctors bring their expertise in medicine and their management of personnel and communication skills to the organization and administration of a healthcare system and a hospital. Their leadership in ensuring the best care for patients in a pleasant environment that is fiscally sound is a great contribution to the profession and healthcare in general.

Professional organizations can benefit from the leadership skills of a physician who will strive for the protection of the highest standards of the profession. Other physicians become leaders in the public health arena, working to ensure the health and safety of the broader community, both nationally and internationally. Their efforts protect our nation's health while having an impact on others worldwide. Similarly, physicians can provide their leadership on the local level of their community or their state.

They can lend assistance to the local public health personnel by gaining community support for necessary health protection actions. They can also assist local and state legislatures in understanding health-related issues of legislation.

Researchers in clinical medicine, whether at university settings or pharmaceutical companies, provide leadership in the development of new techniques, drugs, and medical equipment. Their leadership skills are the force behind the innovation in medical practice and patient care that moves the profession of medicine forward.

All of these leadership positions in medicine ensure quality in the treatment of patients and the working efficiency of our healthcare institutions. Physicians cannot practice medicine without being leaders. Their role as patient advocates demands leadership. *How So?*

A Legacy of Excellence

Considering the best advice I ever received reminds me of how lucky I was to grow up with two physicians in the family. My father and grandfather, both doctors, set standards for me by their example. My grandfather visited his patients on horseback, assuring them the care and attention they required. My father told me doctors work on Saturdays, which I initially didn't think necessary. But I soon learned in medical school and in my practice that keeping abreast of the latest in medicine and being available for patients more often than not requires working on

Saturdays. I did have to acknowledge to my dad that he was right: Doctors work on Saturdays.

no pride here!

With these examples of great doctors in my family, and my own efforts in working to be a great doctor, I find medicine is my life. It is not only an intellectually stimulating but also a demanding profession that requires continuous study and research. Working to be a great doctor requires the practitioner to want to contribute to the art and science of medicine and actually be a part of its future.

And keeps you at constant arms length from, and elevated way above, the peons.

While these thoughts and endeavors are motivating forces in my life and in the lives of many physicians, the practice of medicine is a humbling experience. Our patients' well-being depends on our knowledge, skill, and caring. It is the seriousness of this responsibility that in turn motivates me to work toward excellence. It is the circle of intellectual stimulation, motivation, and humility that brings life to the practice of medicine. *?*

Both my father and grandfather believed and practiced medicine based on the standard that the patient always came first. They told me how putting myself in the patient's place would help me work and live by the standards I had set for myself. "Work to be excellent" was their advice to me. Their standards, their lives, and their practice of medicine are the best advice I could have received from anyone. I believe their example is a model for all physicians in the practice of medicine.

Good Doctor Versus Great Doctor

A doctor who gives a limited number of patients (according to his or her abilities) good care is a valuable asset to the community and the profession, but more is required to be a great doctor. A great doctor is one who influences the pathways of medicine, contributing alternative and innovative ways for better treatment of patients. A great doctor is a steadfast worker and an overall renaissance person who seeks solutions to the many challenges of medicine and healthcare in general.

a great doctor is GOD!!

A great doctor will have an impact on medical education and on the training of interns and residents he or she comes into contact with. A great doctor will keep up-to-date on medical information, attend continuing education programs, and know when to consult. A great doctor will have an effect on the health of the community, sharing experience and knowledge with community leaders. This ability to effect policy change will also be felt at the administrative and board levels of the hospital.

The nature of medicine and its responsibilities sets the physician apart from other professionals. The golden rules for the physician as a person and professional are those of the highest moral and ethical standards. The physician must be ever mindful of the vow to "Do no harm." I pass on to all doctors the advice I received from my grandfather and father: Put the patient first, and put yourself in the patient's place for better understanding.

yeah. It keeps him from being human.

But of course, you yourself will never ever be an actual patient, because you're special + cannot

Doctors face many challenges today, but medical practice remains a rewarding life for the curious, the innovative, the compassionate, and the dedicated.

Dr. W. Randolph Chitwood, Jr., is from Wytheville, Virginia. He completed his undergraduate studies at Hampden-Sydney College and received his M.D. degree from the University of Virginia. He did his residency in general surgery and his cardiothoracic training at Duke University. He became a full professor and Chief of Cardiothoracic Surgery at East Carolina University immediately upon completion of his surgical training. He was named Chairman of Surgery at East Carolina University in 1996.

Dr. Chitwood is a Fellow of the American College of Surgeons and a member of the Society of Thoracic Surgeons and the American Association of Thoracic Surgery. He is currently President of the International Society for Minimally Invasive Cardiac Surgery and President-Elect of the Society for Heart Valve Disease. Dr. Chitwood specializes in minimally invasive mitral valve surgery and performed the first total mitral valve repair with a surgical robot in the United States.

One of the most grandiose piles of self-importance I've ever read !!

et sick, ever..

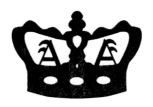

THE GOOD SOUL:
COPING WITH CHALLENGES
FACING DOCTORS TODAY
AND TOMOROW

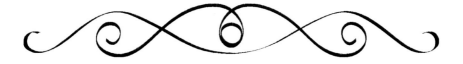

LAURA FISHER, M.D.
The New York Hospital
Internal Medicine & Infectious Disease

Attending Physician

Art, Science, and Obsession

The science of medicine refers to an immense and ever-growing fund of knowledge that describes the normal and abnormal function of the human body. However, medicine is not a pure science, such as physics or mathematics, because no two patients are alike in how they experience (feel the symptoms of) or manifest (show the signs of) an illness. I like to view the individual patient as the canvas and the interacting elements of his or her physical and mental wellness and pathology as the pigments of paint on that canvas. The art of medicine is evident when the individual doctor uses his or her personal experience, intuition, skill, and knowledge to diagnose and improve the physical and mental health of that individual patient.

A medical student must first take basic science courses (such as anatomy, histology, embryology, physiology, and molecular biology) to establish the groundwork for more advanced clinical courses. The rigor of medical studies also trains the student of medicine to think in a logical, deliberate, and systematic manner. The student must have a solid understanding of the mechanisms of wellness and disease before he or she can memorize and use long lists of signs, symptoms, and differential diagnoses. The clinician's responsibility is to further master the science or building blocks of medicine *(e.g.,* cardiology, hematology, dermatology, allergy and immunology, rheumatology, infectious diseases, pulmonary medicine, gastrointestinal disease, oncology, psychiatry, nephrology, neurology, endocrinology) to diagnose and treat the patient correctly. The art of medicine lies in knowing how to retrieve and integrate a seemingly infinite number of possibly relevant facts when encountering a particular patient. This art is demonstrated by the ability to obtain a relevant medical, family, and social history and to perform an accurate and thorough physical exam to make a rapid and proper diagnosis and to devise an appropriate treatment plan.

A doctor must know which questions to ask and how to ask them of a patient in a respectful and non-threatening way. He or she must also know how to interpret a patient's subjective complaints and concerns in light of that patient's social, physiological, psychological, and cultural make-up.

Different patients might have the same underlying disease process, such as angina, yet present with very different complaints, such as chest pain, lightheadedness, shortness of breath, or gastrointestinal upset. Other patients might present with the same complaint – a cough, for instance – yet have different causative illnesses, such as asthma, infection, pulmonary embolism, cancer, or gastrointestinal reflux. A complaint of headache could indicate meningitis, migraine, sinusitis, temperomandibular joint syndrome, temporal arteritis, subarachnoid hemorrhage, or a simple tension headache. Appreciating these varying presentations in different patients relies on the diagnostic art within medicine.

The job of a good internist overlaps with that of a psychiatrist. A clinician must appreciate the interaction of the psyche and the body. He or she must be able to recognize and diagnose psychiatric illness. Many internists feel comfortable prescribing medications for uncomplicated depression and/or anxiety. For example, a new patient presented to me with complaints of headaches, memory loss, shortness of breath, paresthesias, migratory body aches, fatigue, and lightheadedness. She had already been evaluated by several other physicians and had undergone extensive and expensive diagnostic testing; yet no diagnosis had been made and no therapy offered. After a long conversation with the patient, we were able to identify her sense of being overwhelmed by a recent move to New York because of her husband's job change, the recent birth of her first child, and some marital strain. She was actually relieved by the diagnosis of depression and somatization and responded quickly to appropriate antidepressant medication and behavioral therapy.

The art of medicine can also be demonstrated in the effective handling of a patient's phone question. Even without examining the patient, a working diagnosis can often be entertained if one knows which initial and subsequent questions to ask and if one not only listens to, but successfully understands the patient's replies. Recently a patient telephoned because of a rash. By questioning the patient about the color, size, pattern, and location of the rash and of associated paresthesias, I suspected the patient had Varicella Zoster. The patient came in to my office, and appropriate antiviral therapy was initiated. Similarly, a patient might page a doctor at night with the complaint of chest pain. Only a good doctor could relatively accurately distinguish musculoskeletal pain (which could be treated with anti-inflammatory medication and evaluated the next day) from more serious processes, such as pulmonary embolism or ischemia (which would require immediate emergency room evaluation).

Basic or clinical researchers are both scientists and artists, as well. They must have an overwhelming personal passion and vision to ask the proper question and to formulate their hypothesis. An AIDS researcher must first master all of the available scientific facts relevant to HIV infection to then create a new model or laboratory technique or antiretroviral compound. The physician-researcher must be obsessed with a dream – to prevent or cure diabetes, breast cancer, lung cancer, cardiovascular disease, Alzheimer's Disease, epilepsy, or autoimmune disease, for example. His obsession is not unlike that of the greatest artists or poets.

A Good Soul

Good doctors have to be intelligent, diligent, well read, and caring. The main drive for doctors should be that they truly want to help others achieve mental and physical health. Kindness is a prerequisite for good doctoring. Physicians must know how to deal well with people of all ages and of different cultural, ethnic, socioeconomic, and religious backgrounds. As already mentioned, they have to know which questions to ask of which patients and the proper manner in which to ask them. They must be able to listen to and interpret the patient's answers. Physicians must be able to deal with subtleties in physical findings and in patient's complaints. Different patients have different perceptions of pain, shortness of breath, pruritus, and so on. So intelligence, compassion, a strong fund of knowledge, and good detective work (knowing how to put symptoms and signs and risk factors together to find the right diagnosis) are all critical factors in a doctor's success.

Only when a doctor-patient relationship is based on respect, caring, trust, and understanding is the art of medicine clearly demonstrable. A doctor's bedside manner is of the utmost importance in his being an excellent physician, because it invites the patient's necessary participation in the medical process.

I believe the ability to achieve personal and professional success is something most of us begin to establish in childhood. Someone who is happy and well-adjusted in childhood and the teen years will probably remain content, well-rounded, capable, and optimistic in later life. Professional and personal successes usually go hand in hand. If one is personally successful – meaning that one is content with oneself, happy with his or her life circumstances, interested in what he or she is doing, and has strong significant relationships with a husband, wife, family members, or friends – it will be easier to be a good doctor. A doctor's patients, colleagues, and staff will respond to his or her charisma, warmth, and self-confidence. Patients will find it easier to confide in and trust that kind of doctor. Optimism and good will are contagious. Likewise, if the doctor is successful at work – meaning she feels good about her interaction with patients and staff, her ability to help her patients, and her reputation among colleagues and patients, she will take this feeling of contentment home at the end of the day. Family and friends will share and benefit from these good feelings. Conversely, love for family and friends can overflow and manifest as good will toward her patients.

Organizational skills are very important, as well. It is not easy to maintain a stable and happy home life and to have a thriving practice. To succeed at home and at work, one must have excellent organizational and time management skills. Many of the best doctors are married, in a significant relationship, or enjoy significant friendships. They have to multitask. They have to learn how to juggle their personal and professional lives. I am a mother of three young daughters. I have a lot to manage each day between spending precious time with my husband and daughters, supervising a busy household, and running a very busy full-time private practice. My typical day starts around 5:30 in the morning, when our middle daughter awakens. After spending several hours with my husband and daughters, I spend a full and hectic day at the office. I find it beneficial to exercise daily at the gym before returning home. I find that my hour on the stationary bike allows me time to unwind, clear my head, read my beloved novels, and catch up on reading medical journals. I then enjoy spending the evening with family or friends.

There is not much free time available to sleep, catch my breath, or just think. Luckily, I have always had a lot of energy, a sense of can-do, good organizational skills, discipline, and the ability to enjoy almost anything I choose to do. Despite the lack of enough hours in a day, it is important to challenge and reward oneself in extracurricular areas, be they music, art, literature, travel, the theater, or sports.

Countless seminars offer advice on how to be kinder to patients, how to comfort patients, how to respect their confidentiality, and how to give a patient bad news (such as in imparting a cancer or an AIDS diagnosis). However, if one is a good, honest, and kind person, these skills should come naturally. I believe a good soul will manifest itself both at home and in the office.

Face-to-Face is Best With Patients

My strategy for dealing with patients is relatively old-fashioned. I prefer face-to-face contact whenever possible. When a patient calls with a complicated question or problem I ask him or her to come into my office to talk in person. The physician-patient encounter is very important and subject to nuances of a facial expression, a pause or hesitation in conversation, and changing body language. Subtle messages or clues to the patient's psychological state might be lost with a phone conversation, e-mail correspondence, or messages relayed by a nurse, a secretary, or an answering service. Avoidable mistakes are often made when a physician tries to make too many diagnoses or to prescribe therapy over the phone. I have seen cases of appendicitis misdiagnosed as gastroenteritis and cases of pneumonia misdiagnosed as the common cold. Some issues can be handled over the phone if the patient cannot come in for an appointment, but direct, face-to-face time is important whenever possible.

Personally, I have not gone the route of e-mail. I have an e-mail address but do not typically share it with patients. I have found it to be useful on the few occasions when a patient lives in another time zone (making it difficult for phone consultations during office hours) or when consultants have sent me digital photographs of patients' rashes. Just this week I received very helpful photographs of a patient's skin lesions from a referring doctor. One photograph was of the erythema migrans lesion of early Lyme disease, and the other was of recurrent erythema multiforme of unknown etiology. Unfortunately, a lot is lost in translation when people are typing answers and questions back and forth.

Just as you might sip a new wine and know instinctively that it is a good vintage, there are some innate characteristics of a good physician. His or her intelligence and enthusiasm are readily apparent. The best doctors are usually bright, quick-thinking, perceptive, and directed. As I have pointed out, they know how to ask the right questions and can integrate information very quickly and accurately. Typically, they can make the proper diagnosis with fewer tests and procedures and can select the therapy with the most efficacy and the fewest unwanted side effects.

Greatest Challenges Facing Today's Physicians

For the individual clinician, the most basic and common daily challenge is in establishing and maintaining a good patient-doctor relationship. This rapport can be especially difficult to establish with certain patients who might be angry, hostile, frustrated, or frightened. This challenge would be true of any interaction between strangers meeting for the first time.

There are rare occasions when upon first meeting a new potential patient, I am struck by the instinctive realization that the patient is extremely antagonistic or hostile or convinced he or she has an illness that he or she clearly does not have. On these occasions I believe I cannot in good faith take on that patient's care. I have found it is better to explain to that patient that the two of us will, for whatever reason, not be able to establish a therapeutic relationship, and to terminate the intake interview without billing the patient. It is important to explain that this action is in the patient's best interest.

The typical first doctor-patient encounters will bear fruit, however. Trust has to be established and solidified over time. The patient has to be willing to confide in the doctor and has to be willing to answer the doctor's questions honestly. The physician cannot make a diagnosis or determine the correct treatment if he or she does not know the right questions to ask or if the patient does not feel comfortable giving honest and complete answers. A patient must feel at ease in discussing prior or current drug or alcohol use, sexual practices, lifestyle aspects, contraception, dietary preferences, bowel habits, etc. This trust takes time and effort to establish.

On a more macro scale, there are unfortunately countless bureaucratic challenges a doctor encounters. Managed care limits a doctor's autonomy in ordering diagnostic tests, prescribing medication or other types of therapy, and referring patients to outside consultants. Frequently a patient wants to have a mammogram done by an in-network radiologist, while the best mammographers might be out of network. A patient might ask to be referred to a participating surgeon, while the better surgeon might be out of network, as well. Unfortunately, the third-party role of insurance companies can threaten the trust and respect and rapport between patient and physician.

Physicians are often challenged by the allocation of limited resources. Many patients cannot afford the best medications for their conditions. There are frequent shortages of many vaccines. This past year witnessed temporary shortages of diphtheria-tetanus vaccine, Hepatitis B vaccine, influenza vaccine, and Varicella vaccine.

Waitlists for organ transplants continue to lengthen. A just and pragmatic way of distributing these resources must be found. Other ethical issues, such as when it is proper to withhold or discontinue potential life-supporting care, continue to challenge us.

We are witnessing new diseases that must be addressed aggressively and quickly. AIDS was only recognized in the early 1980s and continues to be a major health issue worldwide. Significant work is being carried on regarding prevention and treatment, but an effective vaccine or cure is nowhere in sight. Newer challenges include the crisis with bio-terrorism. What we once thought was merely a theoretical threat was proved a reality when anthrax-infected letters were sent through the United States mail system. We are concerned about the risk of broader bio-terrorism, including smallpox, plague, and the hemorrhagic viruses. Most of us didn't envision such a scenario before the events of September 11th and subsequent weeks.

A doctor must have a consistent and successful approach when encountering a diagnostic roadblock. Interns, residents, and fellows are expected to avail themselves of text books when they are challenged and to seek the advice of more senior physicians at the hospital when the approach they have embarked upon fails. As an internist I prefer having a copy of important reference books both in the office and at home in case of nighttime or weekend calls from patients. When I have difficulty with a particular case, I go back to the beginning and sometimes find clues I missed on first perusal. At this point in my career I am very fortunate to have a terrific list of specialists in other fields whom I respect and whom I can call on for advice when necessary. Sometimes a phone call will answer the question, but it is often necessary to refer my patient for a consultation. I believe the best doctors are those who recognize their strengths, but also acknowledge their limitations. It is important to admit when one doesn't know the answer and to seek that answer elsewhere.

Some doctors use the Internet to get information when they hit a roadblock. From my limited experience, in terms of useful medical information, the Internet offers more breadth than depth. That is fine for physicians at an early stage of training who want to find a wide differential diagnosis or symptom complex list. Unfortunately, I have been disappointed thus far in my efforts to find detailed information on esoteric medical subjects. I prefer referring to the standard medical periodicals, such as *New England Journal of Medicine, Annals of Internal Medicine, Journal of the American Medical Association, The Medical Letter,* and *Morbidity and Mortality Weekly Report.*

The Future of Medical Practice

One of the biggest changes in medicine has already set in, and that is managed care. Individual doctors have already accepted its reality and have decided they either will or will not participate with managed care companies. Although there may be policy changes regarding physician referrals and coverage of diagnostic tests, therapeutic procedures, and prescription medications, I do not believe that managed care will ever disappear.

Electronic information will continue to have an impact on the practice of medicine. A small percentage of physicians are already communicating with their patients online. Again, I am fairly averse to that practice and am not thrilled so far with the communications going on between doctors and patients online. The idea of patients seeking information online before coming to a physician is theoretically good, but thus far I have mostly seen undesirable ramifications. Many a patient has done his or her own computer research and made an incorrect diagnosis. I have seen too many patients who have convinced themselves that they have sero-negative Lyme disease despite the lack of any risk factors or physical findings of Lyme disease. For the physician, it is often difficult to dissuade a patient from an erroneous diagnosis that he or she has made based on online searches. On the other hand, it is often useful for the physician to refer his or her patient who has a definite medical diagnosis to specific physician-approved online sites for in-depth information or advice. Excellent online sites already exist for patients with diabetes, obesity, migraine headaches, epilepsy, sleep apnea, lupus, rheumatoid arthritis, coronary disease, cancer, asthma, hypertension, and countless other illnesses. In the future more electronic medical information will be available to patients. I hope it will be more accurate and accessible and less of a stumbling block when it comes to patients seeking appropriate diagnostic and therapeutic information.

New information regarding disease processes, therapy, epidemiology, risk factor modification, and medical technology is constantly being published. The physician is faced with new diagnostic tests, such as electron beam CAT scans for cardiac calcium scores, whole-body CAT scans for the diagnosis of cancer, PET scans, SPECT scans, thin-prep PAP tests, new breast imaging modalities, blood tests for genetic predisposition to certain cancers (such as BRCA1 and 2), and blood tests for ovarian, breast, prostate, and colon cancers. He or she must be familiar with the ever-growing number of antibiotics, antihypertensive medications, antidepressants, and lipid-lowering agents. A good doctor must read voraciously to keep abreast of this new information. It is important to read journals in general medicine and in one's particular subspecialty as they are released. Much important and useful medical and health-related material can also be gleaned from lay publications, such as *The New York Times* or *The Wall Street Journal.* Doctors must make every effort to attend conferences offered at their hospitals or offered by state and national medical organizations.

Unfortunately, ours is a very litigious society, and countless inappropriate and frivolous malpractice cases are being brought against good physicians and hospitals. So many of these lawsuits are brought by angry or unhappy people looking to lay blame where it does not exist. Certainly there have been valid claims of negligence and medical malpractice, but too many innocent physicians are sued because of misplaced anger, misunderstanding, and greed. Our society must recognize that bad things can happen to good people, and that many bad health outcomes are not preventable. I believe our fear of death and our unrealistic expectations of near-immortality are partly responsible for people failing to understand that not all disease and death can be prevented. Our society often sees promises in medicine where these promises do not and cannot exist. Another atrocity that must be addressed and corrected is the utterly fantastic settlement amounts that juries often determine. I question our current jury system's ability to fairly adjudicate malpractice cases and to determine settlement amounts. I believe a panel of respected physicians and judges would be more able to make decisions in malpractice cases than a lay jury.

Highest Standards

To be a good doctor, one must be kind, hardworking, compassionate, intelligent, and ethical. My six siblings and I learned this lesson from our father, who was and is a great physician of the old school. Each of us chose to become a physician in turn. Our mother is brilliant and talented and would have chosen to enter the medical profession herself had her parents supported her desire at the time and not been convinced that a woman's place was not in medicine. (Thank goodness women are now welcome in medicine.) She obtained her Ph.D. in biophysics and enjoyed a rewarding career in teaching. Both of our parents emphasized the overriding importance of knowledge. We were encouraged to help others in whatever ways we were most capable. In our family the combination of academic excellence and concern for others led to the pursuit of careers in medicine.

Good doctors must be humble, yet confident. They must respect their patients, their staff, and themselves. They have to trust their knowledge base, understanding of and rapport with patients, diagnostic and therapeutic ability, and instincts. They must feel comfortable in making decisions and then take responsibility for these decisions. They must be able to recognize and admit their mistakes and act to remedy these mistakes. They must be open-minded and creative in making an initial differential diagnosis, but insightful and deliberate in honing that differential to a single diagnosis.

Physicians must abide by the golden rule, which is to "love thy neighbor as thyself." The reason we pursue a career in medicine is not for money, fame, or pride, but to help others. Maimonides was a 12th century physician, rabbi, and philosopher whose Prayer for the Physician I like to quote:

> Before I begin the holy work of healing the creations of your hands, I place my entreaty before the throne of your glory that you grant me strength of spirit and fortitude to faithfully execute my work. Let not desire for wealth or benefit blind me from seeing truth. Deem me worthy of seeing in the sufferer who seeks my advice – neither rich nor poor. Friend or foe, good man or bad, of a man in distress, show me

only the man. If doctors wiser than me seek to help me understand, grant me the desire to learn from them, for the knowledge of healing is boundless.

Dr. Laura Fisher received BA degrees in biology and biomedical ethics from Brown University in 1981. She received her medical degree from Brown Medical School in 1984. She was a medical resident at The New York Hospital (Cornell Medical College's teaching hospital) before doing her Infectious Disease fellowship at The Massachusetts General Hospital in Boston. Dr. Fisher returned to be Chief Medical Resident at The New York Hospital in 1989 and has been an attending physician in the Internal Medicine and Infectious Disease divisions there since. She has a private medical practice on the Upper East Side of Manhattan.

Dr. Fisher has been consulted frequently as a medical expert on television (ABC, NBC, CBS, FOX, CNN, and CNBC), on the radio, in newspapers (The New York Times and other regional papers), and in journals (Redbook, Elle, and others).

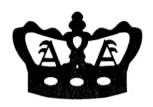

RECAPTURING THE CALLING OF MEDICINE

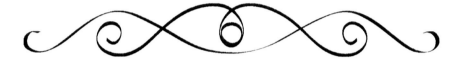

MICHAEL J. BAIME, M.D.
University of Pennsylvania School of Medicine
Penn Program for Stress Management

Director

Art and Science: Defining the Differences

Being a successful doctor involves practicing a discipline that is both an art and a science. The first aspect of that discipline is the discipline of the science of medicine – that is, the ability to skillfully apply medical science and technology to enhance health. This is what we usually think of as the practice of medicine. This aspect truly is a science, as it involves knowing how to change the biology and physiology of the body, and, in particular, how to carefully alter biology to restore health when disease has interrupted and affected it. But there is more to the practice of medicine. The other essential component of being a doctor is the art of healing people – the skill with which the healer can use his or her presence and relationship with someone to make a difference. Although physicians spend most of their time and energy working to master the science of medicine, it is the art of medical practice that provides the deepest satisfactions.

I aspire to combine this art and science as seamlessly as possible. The technical expertise – the science of medicine – is relatively straightforward, even though the amount of information is overwhelming. After all, information is just information. It is objective and concrete, and you can always look it up again if you forget. You remember what you can, and you learn to find the rest when you need it. This has become easier as computer and information technology have made medical information more accessible. Fifteen years ago I spent hours each week keeping a file of journal articles up-to-date. Now I log on to my institution's online library. I have a lot more room in the file drawers in my office. Soon I expect to have access to that information from a wireless digital computer I will carry in my pocket. I already carry a medical textbook and a database of drugs in my pocket organizer. So, although we will always respect the physician who seems to have mastered the immense fund of medical knowledge by remembering the most information, the actual memorization of this knowledge seems to be progressively less meaningful. This is an exciting development, and the use of information technology will continue to reshape the future of medicine in unpredictable and startling ways.

Despite this fabulous technology, however, physicians still need to work very hard to remain abreast of the science of medicine. There is an increasing emphasis on "evidence-based" medicine, which is the practice of medicine based on research and objective data, rather than opinion or belief about how something should be done. One would hope that this is how medicine has always been practiced, but when we actually look closely, we find our beliefs and prejudices may distort our perception of what we actually know. Medical science is working to derive objective guidelines and principles to direct the technical practice of medicine. Getting expertise in that, again, is quite straightforward. But all of the information in the world will not help us be better doctors unless we can take its content, understand how that information applies to each individual patient, and use it effectively. Truth, or at least the truth of medical knowledge, does not stand still. There may, somewhere, be an absolute truth, but in the practice of medicine, all truths are relative. Our knowledge about how to help bodies heal and how to prevent disease is always provisional and in constant flux, just like everything else in the 21st century. People who practice medicine are required to keep up with that constantly changing science. Technology does help by providing access to information, but that information still needs to be processed, evaluated, interpreted, and used to attain a goal.

There is really no easy or practical way to keep up with this constantly rising flood of information. I make an effort to read at least one new article pertaining to my field of internal medicine each day. Doing so allows me to keep pace with the flow of science. Of course, the actual reading of a medical report is not difficult and can be done very quickly. But it can take hours of contemplation and study to actually understand what that article means, to see its strengths and weaknesses, and to appreciate how it applies to one's clinical practice and individual patients. I would like to claim that I always complete this task, but I do not. I am lucky enough to be in a large teaching institution with a teaching practice that has students, interns, and residents working beside the faculty each day. That environment gives me a tremendous number of opportunities for learning, right at my fingertips. Then I do my best, and at the end of each day, I hope my best was good enough. It is a humbling experience to perform a task that so dramatically affects the life of another human being, and to acknowledge that one's mastery of that task will always be incomplete.

The biggest challenge of medicine, however, is not mastery of the information that comes from books. It is mastering the more human aspect of healing, and merging that healing role with the scientific and technical expertise. Physicians need to do this deliberately and proactively. Often we take that part of medical practice for granted, thinking the wisdom of our accumulated experience is enough. Sadly, it often is not. And although the over-emphasis on the science of medicine at the cost of the practice of its art deprives our patients of something they want desperately, the greatest loss is our own. That is because the greatest rewards of medical practice are found in its most human interactions.

We must deliberately cultivate the interpersonal part of healing alongside the technical expertise. It is hard to say exactly how to do this for a particular physician. It is very personal. It is much easier to prescribe a daily medical journal article. I like to think I make both of those aspects a priority and value both equally. It is very difficult to maintain that balance, and it sometimes seems that people who practice medicine tend to be biased one way or the other. It is very common to find that the real technical expert in a field, or the person who is most widely known or most knowledgeable about a particular problem, is the least skillful at the interpersonal art of healing. A cynic might conclude that once they know that they are a real expert, they believe they no longer need to work so hard at caring and feeling. More likely, they are just too busy. In any case, their patients feel their absence, although if most people had to choose, they would choose the doctor with the technical expertise and hope they will get the time and the caring from someone else.

Encouraging Mindfulness

The role of the doctor is to apply technology skillfully and to cultivate his or her inner resources and those of the patient. This is a powerful way to promote wellness and to help the patient heal. It is also very challenging. Part of the difficulty comes from the intense time pressure and stress of current medical practice. We will have to do something to make the practice of medicine less pressured for both ourselves and our patients if we are to continue to provide optimum care.

Here! here!

One way I try to work toward this goal is to teach patients and healthcare providers mindfulness and meditation practices. I run a mindfulness meditation-based stress management program at the University of Pennsylvania, where I teach both patients and doctors to use the concept of "mindfulness" as a tool for healing. This mindfulness is defined as a moment-by-moment awareness of what is happening right now, in each moment. Mindfulness mediation is a technique that teaches one to bring awareness to the present moment and let it remain and rest there. When we remain in the present moment, we find we can relax fully and deeply in that moment. We do not need to worry about what has happened and is already finished or about what is still off in the future and may never occur.

Be here now

LIVING IN TRUTH?

When we begin to notice what our minds are actually doing as we go about our business, it is shocking to find that we are seldom paying attention to what we are doing right now. What doctors usually do when they are with a patient is to carry on numerous different conversations in their heads at the same

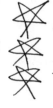

YES! YES! YES!

time.) We are always talking to ourselves, and it is sometimes shocking to see how many different simultaneous conversations we carry on. We tend to do this automatically, on "automatic pilot." This is similar to what happens when we drive home and do not really notice what we are doing, where we've been, what we've seen. When we arrive and get out of the car, sometimes it seems that someone else must have done the driving. We were not paying attention to where we were going at all and don't remember how we got home.

This automatic pilot is not a problem if we are doing something that doesn't matter. It is fine to drive your car on automatic pilot, at least when the ride is uneventful. It is not, however, such a good way to practice medicine, even if we perform the technical aspect of our practice perfectly.

Our absence in the encounter with a patient deprives them of our presence. It is this presence that actually provides a bridge between healer and patient. That one-on-one presence of a doctor, the healer, in the room, making an active, living connection with the patient is what gives that patient a link to themselves, to their own being, to their own heart, and to their own sources of strength and healing. The actual felt presence of that other person is what lets the patient know that someone is there. *This guy gets it!!*

Mindfulness also provides a powerful set of tools for stress management. The ability to rest in the present moment helps people undo their anxiety and face their challenges with balance and confidence. Mindfulness is about learning how to connect with one's own inner resources. My public program at the University of Pennsylvania Health System has trained more than 2,000 people to use meditation as a tool for healing. I also teach classes at the University of Pennsylvania School of Medicine for students and trainees, as well as doctors in practice, to help them use these techniques in their own professional lives and to enhance healing.

Meditation may or may not become more popular, but something that accomplishes these goals is absolutely necessary. It is absolutely necessary for us to come to our senses and reassess the role of our own presence in the art of healing. Without it, a part of what is most important about medicine will remain lost to us and our patients.

The economics of healthcare have painted us into a very small corner. The time pressure that everyone in healthcare feels has made the delivery of healthcare mostly a technological exercise. The act of being a doctor can be reduced to the act of writing a prescription and ordering tests. That is partly because there just isn't enough time to do anything else. We are afraid to start a conversation with our patients because we might open Pandora's box and invite a flood of feeling we cannot manage in our cramped schedule. But it doesn't take hours of relating to a patient to actually let them know they are cared for or to feel the healing presence of someone who cares for them. Instead, it just requires a healer whose mind is stable and steady and present in that moment with that patient. It happens in an instant, and it is felt right in that instant. You don't need to do anything. Just be there. *AMEN*

I believe it is possible to train yourself to return to the simplicity of that presence with another person by using mindfulness techniques or something like them. If we don't do it, the profession of medicine will become increasingly focused on the concrete interaction. Medical care will be something like plumbing or electrical engineering. This mechanical aspect of healing does provide the appropriate technological intervention, but it doesn't provide what people are longing for in their hearts. That is why the medical profession is denigrated in our culture right now. The modern practice of medicine disappoints patients, and it disappoints the people who provide the care, as well. The doctors who care most about this kind of caring for people are the most discouraged and are the most likely to leave medicine. We must correct the overemphasis on technology. This does not mean we should use less technology, but rather that healing needs an interpersonal – as well as a scientific – aspect.

The most challenging part about being a doctor is dealing with the increasing time pressure and constraints that are put on physicians. It was different when I began practicing medicine, and it will be different again. When I started, I spent 20 minutes with each patient and had a much more spacious interaction with them. That has changed, and it will change more in the future.

I now have 15 minutes with each patient. Many practitioners have less. Three or four times an hour, someone walks in the door. I have to hear their story, examine their body, make a decision about what is happening to them, explain it to them, tell them what I think they should do, speak to their fears, and allay their concerns. Even just telling someone I must change their blood pressure medication conjures up a very complicated set of feelings, including questions such as: Will they live? With they have a stroke? Will they be able to have sex? And this densely felt interaction occurs four times an hour. For the physician, it's like playing a 60-minute symphony in 15 minutes. Even if you hit all the notes, it doesn't sound right. It is hard to do it well. It seems impossible to do it well 20 times a day. Many of the best doctors feel they are past their limit and can't manage their practices properly. Every day I hear someone say that they just can't do this much and do it well. I see no signs of this pressure abating anytime in the foreseeable future.

Could we just practice medicine without doctors? Could we dispense technology with a machine that would interview the patient, and plug your body into a computer, as you plug your car into the analyzer at the auto repair shop? Sometimes it seems as if doctors are being asked to fulfill that function. It is very unsatisfying. As the time pressure and the demand increase, you are being asked to perform that function more and more quickly. The result is that you get less and less personal satisfaction, and actually perform your job less well.

Our entire culture is changing in the same way that the practice of medicine is changing. There is no reason to think anything will halt the progression to more speed and increasing demand. As our speed increases, and we find ever more efficient ways to do more things at the same time, it will become even more difficult to practice healing in any real and meaningful way. We will become lost to ourselves, adrift in a sea of multitasking and overwhelming demands. Our culture must be cured of its speed, its tendency toward violence, and its materialism. Our culture is a trap set to catch itself. We are on a path that fosters incredible productivity at the expense of the people inside. This will become increasingly obvious.

Unfortunately, you cannot change the direction of a culture by getting on a soapbox and preaching. This kind of change must come from within, from the people whose lives are affected by the speed and tension of their daily lives. We have to take a look at ourselves, at how we live, and ask if this really works for us. We need to ask if our lives are helping us fulfill our deepest needs. People themselves must recognize that they are part of a larger system and that by moving at this pace, they are lost to themselves. Until we come back to ourselves we can't do anything.

The only way to really make effective change happen is to begin with ourselves. We need to take a good, honest look at ourselves and think about what we want and what we can realistically accomplish. In the face of these challenges, first of all, I have developed a tremendous amount of humility. I do the best I can and accept that it is a process of constant growth and learning. Each time I fail, the failure is actually pointing out something I could learn to do better. Second, I cultivate my own presence and my own being in my own practice, deliberately and intentionally, in an ongoing way. I never want to view my practice in a percentage/product way. I am always working to learn about how to be with people and how to care for these people in their own way, in the way that works for them, as best I can. Fortunately, in the practice of medicine we have the potential to provide a tremendous benefit for others. I believe if we just start with the concrete details of our own medical practice, we can affect others in ways that can really make a difference. Then the larger changes will be more likely to happen. Change happens with one person at a time.

Finding Ways to Change

It is not as difficult to make these changes as it might sound. In my own practice I make a very deliberate attempt to pay attention to the whole person. As doctors, our tendency is to focus on the disease. In this mindset the blood pressure is the problem, and the goal of the visit is to make that blood pressure number what is should be. Although that is one goal, it makes the whole practice narrow and limiting if that is the only thing that happens during a visit. To prevent this narrow and mechanical type of medical practice, I use meditation-based techniques in my practice. They allow me to slow down enough to actually feel or experience what is happening with a patient.

You do not have to learn to meditate to use mindfulness as a tool to enhance medical practice. Doctors don't have to shave their heads or wear funny robes instead of a white coat to use these techniques. Mindfulness in clinical medicine is the simple practice of coming back to your personal presence and experience while you are with a patient. It is not all that difficult to do, although if you are not in the habit, it might be very hard to remember to try.

You can experiment with this kind of approach in your own medical practice or job. For instance, as a doctor, you might stop at the doorway of the examining room before each clinical encounter, take a deep breath, feel that breath settle into your body, and rest briefly in the present moment. This will give you a moment of transition, allowing your mind to let go of the thoughts and activity of the last encounter. You might or might not consider this kind of break in the flow of work "meditation," and I don't think it matters. If you practice formal meditation, the major benefit will be that when you have a few seconds to rest in stillness, you are more effective at actually resting. You are less likely to react to the tension and speed of what has come before.

Then, when you enter the door to see the next patient, you can let that moment of mindfulness continue. You can focus all of your attention on the patient for the first 30 seconds of that visit – say, for the duration of three slow breaths. You might ask the patient a simple question, such as, "How are you?" and then simply rest and watch and feel while the patient responds. Usually, the first few moments of the visit contain transitional small talk, devoid of any real content. I ask doctors to use that time to fully place themselves in the moment. Your only goal during these 30 seconds is to have a full and direct experience of the patient, to be completely aware of what is happening to the patient in the largest sense possible. Feel and notice the patient. By doing this, you will be able to actually see the person who is there, instead of continually processing people in an inattentive, automatic way. If you see four people an hour, eight hours a day, for 10 to 20 years, you begin to do it automatically. You are not a bad or uncaring person; you are just a human being. We begin to pay less attention to events that happen over and over. It takes an active process, an effort, to change this.

The experience of the patient is strikingly different when the physician starts a visit like this. The patient notices something is ... different ... about the doctor today. Of course, nothing is really different except that the doctor is actually in the room with them. But patients feel that something special and meaningful has happened. Often they comment on it or ask about it. Surprisingly, the visit is likely to be shorter than usual, possibly because the patient has received what they really wanted right at the start of the visit. Then they can relax, because they feel more confident that they will be cared for.

We live our lives scanning our environment for the things we fear or want. We are always looking at the past or looking toward the future. It is very easy to miss the moment we are actually in. This is a loss in all sorts of ways. Personally, we can be asleep at the wheel of our own lives. We can coast along in the same direction without ever really taking stock of where we are and where we truly want to go. Professionally, it affects how our patients experience our care. The patient is so present and so exposed in so many different ways.

There are many reasons to fear a simple visit to the doctor. First of all, the reason for the visit is usually something frightening. People don't take medicine or visit doctors because they like to. They participate in medical care because they do not want to suffer disability, pain, or death. These are very reasonable motivators, but frightening ones. Then, of course, they are about to have their body examined in a way that transgresses the social boundaries that protect them in everyday life. They may experience guilt or shame or anxiety. Meanwhile, the doctor is also anxious, probably about whether he can get out of the room quickly enough. There is no blame in that, either; it is very difficult to practice medicine on a schedule, on any schedule. People and their problems do not fit neatly into 15-minute blocks. Then the patients who are in the waiting room will be angry if their wait is too long. But because of all of the distractions, it is easy to overlook the very anxious, half-dressed human being who is lying on the examining table, hoping someone will care. It is so easy to disappoint that person. I have done it thousands of times myself.

Everyone is uncomfortable when that happens, and no one gets what they want. My goal is to undo that unhappy event with meditative techniques that help doctors to stop and be present. When you do actually find yourself there, in the moment, what you tend to find is not a disease state or a blood pressure problem that needs to be fixed, but another person. While this statement seems insignificant, it makes a qualitative but very important difference in what is happening in the room. Patients feel the difference. They feel the attention. Doctors feel the difference, too. A day filled with empty, meaningless drudgery can become a day filled with people the doctor cares for and cherishes. It is the same day, but the awareness or attention is focused in a different direction. Doctors can recapture the calling of medicine. And most surprisingly, it doesn't take any more time to practice this way. The doctor and the patient are both already there. It was just the attention, the human contact, that was missing.

Just as in every aspect of our culture, in medicine, the concrete, material aspect has overshadowed the experiential, felt aspect. Re-exposing this felt aspect is essential. It is a constant process of maintaining a complete awareness of all domains in that interaction. The doctor must be completely aware of the physical and cognitive aspects of a patient and have the ability to decide where the patient needs the most help. I give this same advice to my staff, as well. Pay attention. Observe as much as possible. Notice. If you are taking a patient into an examining room to take blood pressure, take the opportunity to acknowledge the patient as a person, rather than an object. It sounds exhausting, but in reality it is not. It isn't physical exercise. It is a mental event. It is relaxation into the present moment with the patient. It is a learned art.

Finding Your Own Path

There is no prescription for success. The interesting thing about practicing medicine is that it gives you so many ways to find your way as a professional. As with anything that matters, it is important to have clear and explicit goals. However, at the same time, it is important to have some flexibility with those goals. If your goal is to help people, there are numerous ways you can make this happen. Most important, however, is that you follow your own inner voice. You must find a way to make your own way of being fit with what you do. In some cases that might be to relate to people on a very personal level. This is what has sustained me throughout my career. Others will find different ways. I believe the journey toward success in medicine has more to do with finding your own voice and your own path than it does with anything else. It is a deeply personal process. For me, as a clinician, success as a healer or a physician is the ability to simultaneously practice this interpersonal art and to apply the science of medicine.

You must find your own way and live it and trust yourself. My practice is a primary care practice. I used to be the physicians' administrator of a practice. I was the section chief of a division of general internal medicine. I was a leader, and that has its obvious satisfactions and stresses. In my current practice, however, I am just another clinician. Most of my time and energy go toward developing the meditation-based stress management program. I used to practice the meditation on the side, in my own time, and at times it looked as though the program based on those techniques would never be successful in any external way. But it had its own rewards for me personally, so I trusted that and stayed with it. As a result it has become successful in an external way. I now am part of a large university health system. And while I am not leading a practice, that was not what held the personal rewards for me. Speaking with my own genuine voice in my own way makes the difference. I believe, then, that if you have a passion for something and follow that passion, you will end up speaking with a genuine, authentic voice that others can feel and hear. Your passion might be for research or for some other particular aspect of medicine. It might be outside of medicine. It doesn't matter. If you trust it, you will find your own brand of success. Maybe no one else will notice. If you have really listened deeply to yourself, you will not care.

The practice of medicine is one of the most rewarding and powerful things a person can do. It is an incredible and compelling privilege to touch people physically, spiritually, and psychologically. The capacity to actually decrease patients' physical suffering while helping them find their way through life is incredibly powerful. By cultivating my ability to do this, I feel a deep sense of reward. I enjoy the lives I have touched and the people who have been able to benefit. And in return, as they allow me to share their lives with them, I benefit.

For me, the practice itself has become a way to nurture and cultivate my own life. I feel I have learned something precious and mysterious about life through the practice of medicine. I know what it feels like to be a very old person living alone in despair, or to be a new mother filled with hope. From intimate experiences of so many lives, I feel I have learned something essential about what it means to be a human being, alive, in a body that has the energy of the world coursing through it, a fragile body that cannot live forever. I have learned to be afraid and to have the courage to face my fear, and to be afraid and to not have the courage to face my fear. I have learned so much about what life means through my practice. It is such an incredible path. I would never advise anyone to become a doctor for any of the material rewards the profession offers. They are not worth the struggle and loss they cost. But the spiritual rewards are priceless. In our modern technological medical profession, it is almost suspect to talk about the spiritual rewards of practice. But medicine is a calling, and a calling is always a summons from something higher. It is up to you to decide who or what is calling and how you should answer.

Facing the Challenges

The worst part of being a doctor is disappointing people. Often the system takes us away from the real calling of medicine for financial reasons. Practicing in primary care, you develop an immense amount of humility. When I reach a technical roadblock, things are much simpler: I ask for help. It is easy to become overconfident or to feel that you should be able to do something you can't, but that is really a trap.

The harder situation is to be with someone you really can't help. This is the person who has just heard that he or she has cancer that isn't curable. Doctors must deal with some of the saddest and most bitter experiences of human life. There are structured ways of dealing with these situations as a doctor, in terms of how to present the information to the patient, and so on. However, for myself, I find the most important thing is to not turn away. The temptation is to turn away when we run out of technology to apply. As a doctor, if you accept the premise that you are simply applying the science and technology of healing, then when you are done with administering treatment, you have nothing else to do, and you leave. Instead, you must be present with the patient, no matter how hard it is for you as a doctor. Staying there, not leaving, is the real challenge.

While doctors, for the most part, come into medicine with a tremendous sense of altruism, it is often hard to see this from the outside. Part of the problem is that the doctors are so disappointed in the system that a kind of bitterness gets in the way. There is a tremendous drive to not care so much. Actually, people often view that as a positive thing. They feel opening themselves up too much and caring too much will damage them. I actually don't see anyone who has been damaged by caring too much. I believe it is exactly this caring that allows the profession to renew itself. If we don't have that caring, we have nothing. The caring is the most fundamental basis of healing. If we don't practice it, then we might as well be replaced by a machine that dispenses the right prescription.

I respect doctors who can keep their hearts open and never stop caring. Doing this is tough, but important and necessary. It makes it easier for you, as a doctor, to take a larger view of life. We must all face hopeless situations in our own time and in our own ways. It is just built into our being to experience suffering and sadness and loss. Sometimes it is bitterer than others, but there is something about it that is truly a very human experience. It is really important for me to understand this as I try to get through the process of loss while I do what I must for my patient.

Appreciating this process of loss and the fact that death is inevitable for all of us is actually what gives us the deepest appreciation for the life we have right now. We realize life is fleeting and precious. If anything really matters, it is to live the moment as fully as possible, right now. There is absolutely no guarantee we will get another. Having this deeper sense of the fragility of life leads to the deepest rewards of being a physician. It leads us to find depth and meaning in our work. It teaches us how fragile and precious is this human existence. It transforms the practice of medicine into a path toward a deeper understanding of life itself.

Dr. Michael J. Baime, director of the Penn Program for Stress Management, received his B.A. from Haverford College and his M.D. from the University of Pennsylvania School of Medicine. He completed his residency training in internal medicine at the Graduate Hospital, after which he served as Chief Medical Resident at the Graduate Hospital.

Before joining the Penn Health System, Dr. Baime held a number of administrative positions at the Graduate Hospital, including Assistant Program Director of the Internal Medicine Residency, Director of Ambulatory Services, and Chief of the Division of General Internal Medicine. He is a Clinical Assistant Professor of Medicine at the University of Pennsylvania School of Medicine and is a Diplomate of the American Board of Internal Medicine. His special interest is stress management, and he runs a systemwide program for the University of Pennsylvania Health System. He has been included in

Philadelphia magazine's "Top Doctors" issue for seven consecutive years, including this year's "Top Doctors for Women" issue.

In 1992 Dr. Baime founded the Stress Management Program to address the growing need for the treatment of stress and associated health problems without the use of medications. The program was developed to address the psychological and physical aspects of stress that are difficult to treat in an outpatient practice. More than 2,000 individuals have participated in this public program. In 2001 and 2002 he and his team created and taught two highly successful stress management programs designed to address the needs of healthcare professionals. More than 145 Philadelphia-area doctors, nurses, and other healthcare professionals attended the course.

Dr. Baime has lectured and taught stress management techniques throughout the country, including engagements for the American Medical Association (AMA) and the American Occupational Health Conference (AOHC). He has discussed mindfulness meditation on National Public Radio's "Fresh Air" and has been interviewed for a segment of ABC's "Nightline."

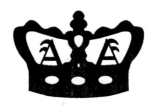

THE PATIENT, PLEASE,
NOT THE DISEASE

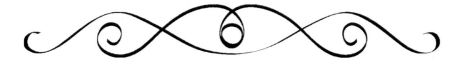

LEO GALLAND, M.D.
MDheal, Inc.

President

The Need for Patient-Centered Diagnosis

For the past 20 years I have had a practice that extends beyond conventional internal medicine. I see people who have chronic and difficult-to-solve problems. My patients range from children with autism to adults with cancer or degenerative neurological diseases. They include people with very well-defined illnesses, such as inflammatory bowel disease and people with much more vaguely defined conditions, such as chronic fatigue.

I was trained in the conventional medical model, which basically holds that people get sick because they get diseases. Each disease is then viewed as an independent entity that can be given a diagnostic code and can have appropriate treatments attached to it. These diseases can be studied in school without reference to any single patient who has the disease.

Over the past hundred years this tendency within conventional medicine has only become stronger and stronger. Today if you are a doctor practicing in the United States and are dependent on any government regulatory mechanisms or third-party reimbursement, you cannot treat a patient unless you attach an ICD (International Classification of Diseases) code to that patient's diagnosis. Furthermore, any treatments you do that are reflected in CPT (Current Procedural Terminology) codes must be appropriate to that ICD code. Thus, the identity of the patient as an individual becomes just a footnote to the disease.

Today we also see the prevalence of evidence-based medicine. This approach to medicine rests on the results of double-blind, placebo-controlled trials. In a double-blind, placebo-controlled trial, researchers treat groups of people with the same disease and try to control for variability among individuals. A basic tenet of this method is that one can remove the inter-individual variability and just look at the treatment for the disease itself. Evidence-based medicine and conventional medicine in general rely on a diagnostic process that asks, "What disease does this patient have?" This is the primary question doctors are first taught to ask and then to answer. The treatment that follows is the treatment for the disease, not necessarily the treatment for the individual. Although medical students hear the adage, "Treat the patient, not the disease," the truth is that doctors don't learn how to treat patients – they only learn how to treat the disease.

After completing my training in internal medicine, I became dissatisfied with the limitations of disease-centered medical practice and began looking for ways to improve the efficacy of medical treatment. I was especially concerned about the long-term outcome for people with chronic or recurrent illness. I called patients I hadn't seen in some time to ask them how they were feeling and what they were doing to take care of themselves. I was constantly impressed by the large degree of individual differences in response to the same kind of therapies. I also realized that an individual's short-term response to treatment was a poor predictor of how well the person would be many months later. For most patients, long-term health status had less to do with the disease or its treatment than with characteristics of the individual, such as family and social support, dietary practices, personal habits, or the environments in which they lived.

I realized that in the evaluation of patients, doctors must analyze those individual factors that contribute to the genesis of illness and to long-term outcomes. I developed a process for organizing and structuring this analysis, which I called patient-centered diagnosis. I apply this process to each individual I work with. I then use this approach to try to generate therapies that are specifically targeted for that individual – therapies that might be quite novel for other people suffering from the very same disease.

Understanding Mediators, Antecedents, and Triggers

The concept of patient-centered diagnosis is as follows. People become ill because of factors I call mediators, antecedents, and triggers, or MAT. It is possible to understand these scientifically. If you can identify the mediators, antecedents, and triggers in each individual case, you can achieve much better results than if you only treat the disease. Knowing what the disease is may give you some idea of what the mediators are, but it often will not tell you about the other factors you must be also aware of.

Mediators

Mediators are not the causes of diseases; rather, as their name implies, they are intermediaries. Mediators are those things that occur to produce the eventual manifestations of disease. Probably the hottest area of medical research in the 20th century involved understanding the chemical mediators of disease underlying both inflammation and coronary heart disease, as well as the spread of cancer. The fascinating thing is that such scientific pursuit revealed that mediators are not disease-specific. That is, these chemical mediators are each involved in multiple diseases, and each individual disease involves multiple mediators. It is possible, then, to understand illness based on mediators without delving too deeply into specific diseases.

Biochemical mediators are not the only kind. Psychosocial mediators, for example, interact with the biochemical mediators in a very direct fashion. Social reinforcement and support, as well as beliefs and expectations, play important roles in mediating the entire phenomenon of illness and disease. It is important, then, for a doctor to look at all of the mediators involved in any one patient situation.

The second thing we must understand is that mediators do not cause disease. Instead, they are part of response patterns that allow organisms to maintain equilibrium in the face of changing or stressful environments. Most conventional drug treatments are aimed at suppressing mediators that have run out of control. We can see this by simply looking at drug category names. We have beta-blockers and calcium-blockers, antihistamines and ACE (angiotensin-converting enzyme)-inhibitors. We have developed an armamentarium of pharmacological substances whose primary action appears to be suppressing hyperactive chemical mediators. The side effects of these drugs are a direct extension of their effects on the body.

Again, mediators are not there to cause disease; they exist instead to regulate the changing environment, internal or external. Numerous factors in a person's life influence the activity of these mediators. Diet and nutrition are important areas I have emphasized in my practice, but there are others. For example, there are natural rhythms – daily, monthly, or seasonal – that have an effect on mediator activity, as well. Understanding how these rhythms affect an individual can be very useful in designing therapies that help prevent relapses.

Triggers

We are exposed to many things internally and externally that can act as triggers for the symptoms of illness. The most obvious example is the person who suffers from allergy and is exposed to an allergen. That person may then develop a skin rash or wheezing. There are many diseases that are not ordinarily considered allergic, in which environmental, dietary, or psychosocial triggers can be identified if the doctor looks hard enough. Helping the person eliminate those triggers can produce improvement, if not a cure.

Triggers must not be overlooked. As an example, let's take a disease called Sjogren's syndrome. This syndrome is an illness that can have very different manifestations, but the hallmark symptoms are dry mouth and dry eyes due to inflammation involving the glands that produce saliva or tears. It appears to be an autoimmune disease. People with this syndrome can have skin rashes and joint pains, and they can experience difficulty with concentration and memory due to inflammation impacting on the brain. There is basically no conventional treatment, except to treat the symptoms. Some studies, however, have indicated patients with Sjogren's syndrome have a tendency to produce antibodies directed against gluten, the protein in wheat. Most of the patients I have seen with this syndrome have benefited greatly by eliminating gluten from their diet. Gluten, in some patients, is basically a trigger for part of the mechanism provoking the syndrome. This, however, is not a specific disease association because many different diseases may be triggered or activated by gluten. Also, gluten sensitivity is not the cause or the only cause of Sjogren's syndrome; it is one factor involved in aggravating it for many individuals.

Antecedents

Antecedents are those things present in the individual, before the onset of illness, which contributed to the illness. There are several types of antecedents, and understanding them is very important in understanding how to proceed with an individual and in getting a handle on the actual prognosis.

There are basically three types of antecedents. First, there are genetic factors. Today a great deal of attention in medical research is being devoted to genetic factors as antecedents in illnesses. However, I believe most of this research is displaced; that is, most of the relationship between genes and illnesses has more to do with the regulation and activation of genes and how environmental influences alter gene expression than it does with gene inheritance. Much of the genetic research will help us understand the chemical mediators of illness better, but – in the short term, at least – I do not think it will shed much light on the antecedents of illness. That is not to say that it won't be able to do so in the future, but for now the attention is overly focused on the notion that genes are the actual cause of the illness. In reality they are just one part of the background of the illness, as antecedents, or rather, as influences on the mediators.

Just as important, we must also look at the events and experiences of the individual patient's life, as these experiences can condition and shape the development of the immune system or the psyche in the direction of illness. Some studies have been done here, as well, especially looking at patterns of childhood abuse as they relate to illness patterns involving the gastrointestinal or reproductive systems in adult women. Again, however, we cannot overgeneralize these results and apply them to each particular patient.

The third type of primary antecedent is the precipitating event. A precipitating event, most simply, is something that happens to a person. Before this event, the person considers himself or herself normal; after this event, however, he or she has become a patient. They now see doctors, and there has been a general change in health and condition.

I then identify this precipitating event, which I do by first asking the patient, "When was the last time you felt perfectly well?" This is a very different question from, "How long have you had this disease?" The answer to the former will lead me back to the antecedents of the illness. Some people have been unwell in one way or another for most of their lives. You must think of these people differently than you think of those who have been perfectly well and have suddenly been struck by illness.

I continue by asking the patient what exactly was going on in his or her life prior to this illness. What things changed? What occurred? The things that turn up are amazing in that they lead to a variety of different and unique approaches to treating the patient.

For example, a disease called ulcerative colitis (an inflammation of the large intestine) comes on in late adolescence or late adulthood. It lasts for life and can be incredibly severe. The symptoms are generally diarrhea, blood in the bowel movements, abdominal pain, fever, and weight loss. Those who suffer from this disease have an increased risk of colon cancer. What amazes me most is that, of the patients that I have seen with a diagnosis of ulcerative colitis, a good 20 percent of them actually have infections as the cause of their colitis.

One way to figure out who is likely to have an infectious colitis and who is not is to look at the origins of the illness. Often people who have traveled extensively to third-world countries have developed an acute diarrheal illness upon their return. The diagnosis of an infectious cause was not considered in these people because the antecedents of the disease were not considered. Instead, the gastroenterologist simply performed a colonoscopy, found what appeared to be ulcerative colitis, and started treating them for ulcerative colitis. This happens less and less these days, but even so, the mere occurrence of it is yet another manifestation of the tendency to look for the disease and make the disease diagnosis, and not look at the actual background of the illness, which often can lead to a different explanation.

Making a Patient-centered Approach Work

The appeal of a disease-centered approach is that it can be adapted into a kind of cookbook, in readily and rapidly applied format. That is: Here are the criteria; you meet the criteria; and these are the treatments that go with the criteria. There is little problem solving, little thinking, and limited data gathering. Advances in healthcare technology may help this system work in some cases, but there is a very large gap between medicine's scientific potential and its actual performance.

Ignoring the role of the individual patient in healthcare undermines the effectiveness of the system. Seventy-two percent of chronic disease and premature death in the United States could be prevented if available medical knowledge were thoroughly applied, but successful application requires an understanding of the individual characteristics of patients, their nutritional habits and lifestyles, and their attitudes and sources of social support. Disease resulting from medical errors and the side effects of prescription drugs has become a serious public health problem, constituting the fourth leading cause of death in the United States. Many adverse drug reactions occur because doctors have neglected the individual characteristics of patients for whom the drugs were prescribed. The conventional, disease-centered model of healthcare fails a lot of individuals, shortchanging the patient, the doctor, and society as a whole.

The first step to a more comprehensive and flexible approach to treating patients lies in accurate and thorough data gathering. By deconstructing an illness using the patient-centered approach, I can then reconstruct different approaches to therapy. To accomplish this goal, I must first gather the data necessary to understand the patient as an individual in relationship to the illness.

Information technology can be very helpful in this area. Huge gains have been made in the application of science and technology to healthcare. The reality is that the way in which data is gathered from patients has not changed in 150 years, and the result is that the process is incomplete. This is an important process because the majority of important information about the patient is still gathered verbally from the patient. However, doctors don't have time to gather all of this data, and even if they did have the time, they would then have trouble organizing it in a useful fashion. Furthermore, often, even if they did have the data organized in a useful way, they might have difficulty deciding how to actually respond to and apply the data.

Although technology has been blamed for the impersonality of healthcare, I believe that information technology – properly applied – can make healthcare more personal and enhance the relationship and communication between patient and doctor. For the past several years I have been working on an information technology approach to patient-centered diagnosis, founding MDheal Inc., an information technology company, in 1999. The way the approach works is that the patient, using computer software, answers a large number of questions, either directly or indirectly through an interviewer. These are detailed questions about symptoms and their characteristics, standard medical questions, family history, diet, lifestyle, social circumstances, and environment. The information is then filtered, reformatted and presented to doctors in a manner in which doctors are trained to see data. Basically, MDheal is a tool designed to facilitate doctor-patient communication.

I envision a future in which computer technology enhances rather than hinders the delivery of personalized healthcare. I believe more personalized care will lower healthcare costs by being more effective and by incorporating individually-oriented strategies for maintaining health and preventing illness. I believe information technology will help patients be more active in their own care and that involving patients in this way will yield better health outcomes. In this vision there is one comprehensive collection of clinical data filled out by *both* patient and doctor and available in digital format and on paper to patients and their physicians. Doctors will enter detailed observations on a handheld computing device while examining the patient. All the data will be automatically transformed into a comprehensive, structured medical record and Problem List.

Each problem identified will be automatically linked to a database for additional information. Therapies based on the recorded characteristics of each individual patient will be retrieved. An expert guidance system will highlight those characteristics of each patient that must be addressed for care to be effectively tailored to the needs of that individual. The system will integrate nutritional, environmental, and psychosocial influences with detailed analyses of symptoms, family medical history, and the patient's own life history. The doctor will be given information that enables an integrated approach to management of the patient's health needs. The patient will receive educational information, instructions for self-managed care, and motivational encouragement that will be automatically generated for each patient, enhancing treatment compliance, patient retention, and treatment outcomes.

Such a program can change the nature of a visit to a doctor. It can create time for more personalized care and give patients more information about their health problems. It can make it possible for patients to receive authoritative advice about new or innovative therapies from their doctors. It will enable doctors to address the needs of their patients more thoroughly and effectively.

We are presently in discussion with some major healthcare centers that are interested in implementing this system. I target the providers of healthcare rather than the third parties. The problem with HMOs and insurance companies is that the way the system is currently organized, employers frequently change insurance companies, as they are constantly looking for better rates. As a result the average person stays with one insurance company for about three years. Because of this, insurance companies are not necessarily interested in long-term cost savings, and instead, they focus on the short-term, bottom-line savings.

We instead target the providers of healthcare systems that have a national or international reputation for high-quality healthcare. We want to start with places that are truly interested in offering the best care they can offer. Our approach has therefore been to go to these providers and explain to them that by using our approach, they can allow their doctors to be more effective and can therefore render higher-quality, more comprehensive service without increasing costs – most likely, with decreasing costs.

In terms of specific demographics we target chronic-care ambulatory patients, not acute care in the hospital. As we have worked through the system, we have ended up focusing on ambulatory patients who are receiving chronic or ongoing care, who speak English, and who are likely to be computer literate, or have access to computers at home.

Once we establish the value of this program and approach in settings where it is easier for it to operate, we will develop foreign-language versions, as well as versions that use perhaps a different vernacular for asking questions. What will need to happen is that health systems will have to allocate space and a certain amount of resources to allow for patients to come in and take the computer interview in the actual facilities. One eventual possibility might be for the entire system to work around a touchtone screen with verbal questioning via headphones. The technology is here; we just presently lack the necessary funding.

In the end my goal is to support healthcare by bringing in this entire dimension that has been squeezed out by technological advances – that is, the communication between doctor and patient, and the body of information that the doctor must have to responsibly and most effectively work with the patient. One hundred years ago doctors made house calls. Doctors knew what a patient's home was like. They knew what kinds of foods they were eating. They could see what the interactions were like with family members. And while this specific interaction almost never happens anymore, the information gained in this venue is absolutely important. Many scientific studies tell us of the importance of this information.

The Healthcare Climate: Two Counteracting Trends

Over the past 30 years I have seen the existence of two distinct currents that have struggled with one another. On the one hand, there is a negative current. There has been an increasing bureaucratization in healthcare. This trend has been based on the reification of disease entities. That has shaped not only education and training, but also compensation and hospitalization practices. As a result it has had an incredibly negative effect on healthcare, on the morale of physicians, and on the satisfaction of patients.

On the other hand, there has been a secondary trend that has taken several forms. The first is an increasingly actively expressed desire on the part of consumers of healthcare not to play a passive role. Consumers are beginning to ask more and more questions. They want to be informed. They want to work in a cooperative fashion with the doctor, not be merely acted upon by the doctor. And while this shift has taken many different forms, there has been an undeniable sea change over the past 30 years in the relationship between patients as consumers and doctors as providers.

Second, there has been a great deal of scientific research validating the importance of knowing the patient's agenda, psychosocial factors, diet and nutrition, and environmental influences in the development of illness and the development of strategies for helping people get better. The kinds of interventions I bring to healthcare are increasingly supported by scientific research, which has been quite gratifying to me.

I advocated things 15 or 20 years ago, based on a relatively small amount of data that made sense to me, that now continuing research has subsequently shown to be important. These include the role of the omega-3 essential fatty acids in the development of illnesses and in the treating of a wide variety of illnesses. I first started lecturing about those in the early 1980s, and the research started to appear in the late 1980s, continuing into this century.

The importance of these fatty acids and the role they play is highly significant. In my book I report the case of a schizophrenic adolescent who had an amazing response to treatment with essential fatty acid therapy. There was a recent double-blind, placebo-controlled trial looking at various fatty acid supplements in treating schizophrenics, which was actually a follow-up to a study done at the National Institutes of Health on patients with manic-depressive illness. It identified the component in omega-3 essential fatty acid therapy as something called EPA (eicosapentaenoic acid), which is beneficial for the treatment of individuals with schizophrenia and very helpful for bipolar disorder, or manic-depressive illness. This was not a substitute for drugs, but it worked so well for manic-depressive patients that the study was stopped six months early because it was clear that one group was doing so much better than the other group, and the researchers said they couldn't go on with the double-blind placebo in good conscience. When they stopped the study, the researchers found it was actually this particular fish oil that was making the difference.

Unfortunately, the government has created and generally continues to foster the first trend. They have encouraged the development of procedures and tests that they will, for the most part, pay for quite readily, while discouraging doctors from spending time finding out what they really need to know about their patients. I don't see this changing. Government is almost never personal, and it is usually pretty stupid. And while there have been a number of initiatives to educate lawmakers, these initiatives tend to be small. Lawmakers understand the system as it is and on its own terms, making the education of these lawmakers a hard task.

The main effects of these initiatives have been attempts to de-stigmatize psychological therapies and to bring them into the mainstream, all of which is helpful. Also, the growing interest in alternative and complementary therapies may help foster a more personal interaction between doctor and patient. One of the reasons people are interested in alternative and complementary therapies is that they tend to be more personally oriented, rather than disease oriented. To the extent that the government supports that, it begins to soften the bureaucracy and increase doctor-patient interaction. Even so, we have a long way to go.

However, aside from these bureaucratic challenges, as well as the inherent difficulty of working with people who have complex, chronic, multifactorial illnesses, there are still more challenges to the doctor. The large amount of new information doctors must understand and apply on a regular basis poses a challenge to doctors today. In this area, information technology can be very helpful. At some point it is my vision to take the kind of patient information gathered by the tools MDheal is developing, and to use that data to generate automatic searches of the new literature databases that are available. In this way, then, with a few mouse clicks a doctor can find relevant information about potential treatments for a patient that are based not only on the disease, but also on the individual characteristics of the patient.

The Science of Caring

In general, doctors who are fresh out of training tend to be at their most arrogant. In hospital training you see patients for only a short period of time. You see them in the acute and critical situations in which the tools that are presently available tend to be the most effective. Young doctors tend not to have had the humbling experience of treating patients over a number of years and seeing those treatments fall apart with relapses of chronic illness. They have not yet discovered that you can do a fantastic job of helping pull someone through a crisis, but not being able to prevent the next crisis.

A number of residency programs are stressing patient-centered approaches and comprehensive approaches to interviewing. However, the studies that have been done have shown no increase in patient satisfaction resulting from interactions from doctors who have been trained this way. It is obvious, then, that things are still being left out.

I believe the reasoning for this is that whenever the educators begin talking about a patient-centered approach within medical education or training, what they really mean is a psychosocial approach. As a result doctors who are trained that way tend to take a strongly psychological approach to chronic illness. Many patients are not interested in that, and whether the patient may be right or wrong, the doctor must certainly have the ability to understand the patient's agenda and not just to impose his or her own agenda.

I have identified a set of necessary skills that I call the Science of Caring. Each of these skills is fundamental to a helpful and successful doctor-patient relationship. They involve the following:

First, the doctor needs to have the ability to actively listen to a patient to try to elicit the patient's story and concerns.

Second, the doctor must have the ability to acknowledge and understand a patient's agenda. Again, every patient has his or her own agenda, and often the true agenda is quite different from what the patient appears to be coming in for. Sometimes these agendas exist in addition to the disease the doctor is treating, and sometimes they are completely distinct. A doctor must be able to understand that to be effective.

Third, the doctor must have the ability to carefully explain things to the patient. If the doctor can't do it, there should be someone in the doctor's office who can. Studies have shown the main thing patients want from doctors is information and explanation. Most doctors tend to think patients just want drugs and a quick fix. But in reality this is not true, and it is becoming less true.

Fourth, the doctor must have the ability to understand the context in which the patient became ill. Here, again, the doctor must look at things like family and social support, environment, and dietary factors.

The first three skills are basic human characteristics that most individuals have the capacity to access if they understand the importance of accessing them and if they have some training in doing so. The fourth requires a fair amount of information and knowledge.

Finally, the doctor must have the ability to show empathy. He or she must know how to offer reassurance, encouragement, and hope to the patient without being deceitful and dishonest.

Studies have shown that 80 percent of premature death and disability result directly from factors related to diet, nutrition, lifestyle, and other alterable life patterns. The biggest challenge in medicine – and therefore its greatest promise – lies in helping patients change those behaviors that cause disease. We need that, and will benefit from it far more than continued work on the genome, for example. I love basic science. I love understanding the basic foundation for the development of illness, and I am glad that further work in this area will continue. But that is not the main thing that is needed now. If the already available knowledge were applied in a thorough manner, we could alter the health of individuals in the county and cut costs far more effectively than any scientific research will help us do, at least in the foreseeable future. This is the change I look forward to.

Dr. Leo Galland graduated with honors from Harvard University, earned his medical degree at the New York University School of Medicine, and completed his training in internal medicine at the NYU-Bellevue Medical Center. He has held a research position at Rockefeller University and teaching positions at the Albert Einstein College of Medicine, the State University of New York at Stony Brook, and the University of Connecticut. He has been in private practice in New York City since 1985. In 1997 he founded the Foundation for Integrated Medicine to foster the integration of nutritional and environmental medicine into clinical practice and medical education. In 1999 he founded MDheal Inc. to develop computer software that enhances doctor-patient relationships and enhances the clinical encounter.

Dr. Galland is internationally known as a pioneer in nutritional medicine and environmental health and as a master educator, clinician, and medical detective. He has extensive experience in developing medical innovations and introducing them to the medical community. Health practitioners and patients throughout the United States, Canada, Europe, and Australia have sought his advice and consultation.

Dr. Galland has appeared as a featured medical expert on ABC, PBS, CNN, MSNBC, Fox Cable Network, the Christian Broadcasting Network, the Trinity Broadcasting Network, and dozens of local affiliates of the major broadcast networks. Interviews with Dr. Galland and articles about his work have appeared in Newsweek, Reader's Digest, Redbook, McCall's, Self, Bazaar, Men's Fitness, Allure, Bottom Line, The New York Times, the New York Daily News, The Washington Post, and many other publications. The New York Daily News listed Dr. Galland among "50 People to Watch in 2000," citing his leadership in developing innovative approaches to healing. He is the author of several dozen scientific publications and two highly acclaimed books that have a special following among health professionals: Power Healing (Random House, 1998) and Superimmunity for Kids (Dell, 1989).

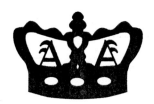

IT'S ABOUT
THE HUMAN BEING

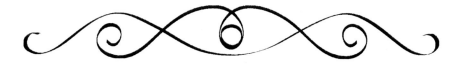

ROSALIND KAPLAN, M.D., F.A.C.P.

The Art of Partnering With the Patient

What we learn in medical school and in residency training – physiology, biology, medications – is basically science. The art, which schools are gradually beginning to teach students, is the spirit of healing. I don't think I was ever really taught that; after medical school, when I became a resident and actually had responsibility for patients in the hospital, I realized I knew nothing about taking care of people. Caring for patients requires much more than merely knowledge of medicine. To really practice the art of medicine, you have to know your patient with a depth that many doctors do not like to get into, because it is very time-consuming. You need to know the history of a patient – not just their medical history, but who they are, what they've been through, what their bodies have been through, and what their minds have been through. Things that happen to us early in life change the whole way our bodies and minds function and react to things. The most important thing is to know your patient.

I also think there is a real art to being able to talk to patients and realize they are human beings. A doctor doesn't look at a disease; a doctor examines a human being. You want to look at the whole person, asking yourself, "How can I help this person have the best quality of life, given any limitations they may have and what their needs will be in the future?" When I add medicine and medical interventions into the art, I ask myself, "How will this affect this person's life? How will it make them feel, emotionally as well as physically?" In many ways, the art lies in being a partner with the patient.

The field of medicine keeps growing with new technology. A doctor needs to keep up with the technology. You need to know what test will get the appropriate information for you, what the differential diagnosis is, and what the possibilities are, based on what the patient describes to you. You need to know what tests are needed, once you know what is wrong with the patient, what treatments are available, and which treatments are most effective for the particular problem. You really do need to know all the science behind that. It is challenging, these days, to keep on top of the game. Every day there's a new medication, and you need to know everything about it – how it interacts with other drugs, and so on.

The difference between the art and the science is that for questions of science, you can look up information in a book – you can pick up a book, go online, or pick up your Palm Pilot, and you can find every drug interaction for every drug that's out from two months ago back. The science of medicine, although there's a tremendous amount of it, is always available if you use resources. Knowing how to find that information becomes a very important skill. The art, however, you have to find inside yourself. Ham

An Alternative Path to Success

My definition of success as a doctor may be different from that of other doctors. I finally feel successful now because I did something a little unorthodox a couple of years ago. I left the group practice I was in, which was part of a health system. The practice had fallen into the trap that all primary care medicine has fallen into now, which is – because of all the discounted insurance and HMOs – that a practice becomes a mill, where it's difficult just to break even in the office, and I don't think we ever did. You have to push patients through at a tremendous rate, and you have to have huge panels of patients. Consequently, I don't think our patients were very happy because everything was very difficult – getting through on the phone, getting appointments – such that they never got the time they needed. The doctors were always in a rush and running late.

The dissatisfaction of my patients made me feel terrible; I think patients should leave an office visit feeling they've had their questions answered. If possible, patients should leave feeling reassured, and if that's not possible, they should leave assured that everything is being done that needs to be done – that if other doctors need to be spoken to, that will happen, or if a follow-up is needed, that will happen, and that the lab results will actually be looked at, and the patient will get a call. The doctor should also take the time to think through each issue and come up with the best possible plan, not just the most expedient one. I think that level of security for the patient has gone by the wayside in many practices.

As a physician, I was exhausted. I was very unhappy. I didn't eat or go to the bathroom some days because I was running from room to room, and it was a very unsatisfying practice. I work with a lot of patients who have deep, complicated problems; I spend a lot of time with eating disorders and other common mind-body problems. When I was unable to spend an appropriate amount of time with a patient, it was truly devastating to the patient. If I did spend enough time with them, I'd spend the rest of the day trying to catch up. So if I actually had a chance to fully deal with a problem, I'd be late for my subsequent appointments and have more and more people angry with me. The staff would say, "You're late! You're late! You're late!" For me, that was not a successful way to be practicing. Some people would have thought I was a very successful doctor then because everybody in the area wanted to come to our practice, especially the women. But in fact I was very unhappy. My kids would tell me I was not home enough, or that they wanted to talk to me about something, and I wasn't there. I also wasn't taking care of myself – that was the biggest downside to that lifestyle. If you can't take care of yourself, you can't take care of your patients. You have to be able to be an example, because if you don't know what to do for your own health, then how can you know what to do for a patient?

Completely unhappy under that system I decided to conduct an experiment. When I told one of our administrators (with whom I'd never gotten along well to begin with, because he wanted to push the patients through, and I would protest), he said, "I've really been thinking about the way you practice, and I think maybe you should try a psychiatric model." Under a psychiatric model, patients pay for time, and most psychiatrists don't take HMO and other discounted insurances – people pay out of pocket. Psychiatrists don't have a lot of overhead because they don't have a lot of staff. I thought it was an interesting concept. In a way, I do practice a lot of psychiatry. But people need medical care, and some of them need the 10-minute visit for the sore throat.

So instead I ran a mixed model: I rented a very small space, hired one staff person who had some nursing background and administrative abilities, and set up three phone lines instead of 10 (one for outgoing calls and two for incoming calls, so people wouldn't get a busy signal). I had a person answering the phone instead of an answering machine that would tell the patients to push option 1, 2, or 3 and then put them on hold for 20 minutes. I allowed half an hour for follow-up appointments and an hour for a physical or if a patient said he or she had a complicated problem and really needed to talk to the doctor. I started out charging what I considered a very reasonable fee for that amount of time. My overhead was low. I didn't take any of the discounted insurances. I did accept Medicare – and still do. As an out-of-network provider, patients could pay up front and then submit the charges to their insurance companies. If I used good documentation of diagnoses and the patients filled out their insurance forms, they would get at least a portion of the costs returned to them. The only kind of insurance this doesn't work for is HMO's, which require the physicians to follow their protocols.

When I started my new practice I thought, "Now I'll just have a few patients. I'll have a tiny practice." Fortunately, I didn't worry a lot about my income at that point because I have a working husband who is also a physician. It turned out that patients loved it. I thought very few patients would come from my old practice, but I ended up with people flocking in because they needed the TLC and the time, and they were willing to pay for it. For the few patients who truly couldn't pay, we worked things out. We bartered for services a few times – I got back equal value of something, sort of like the old model of bartering, where the doctor gets a chicken, and the patient gets medical care.

Living in an affluent area and having a niche with eating disorders and psychosomatic problems put me in a fortuitous situation. The timing was right, and it worked. The practice grew, and I actually got to the point where I felt too busy. As it happened, one of my partners from my former practice wanted to leave that practice to try doing the same thing. So we got a larger space, and we now share an office with two staff people – one is a medical assistant, and one is a receptionist/administrative person – and the four of us run the office. Every phone call gets answered, and every patient gets a half-hour or an hour to meet with one of the doctors. I'm happy. I feel successful. I don't make a lot of money, but I feel successful because I'm practicing medicine the way I want to practice medicine.

There was a recent *Newsweek* article about doctors opening these small practices, and now many people in Boston are talking about "concierge practices," where people pay some amount of money up front, depending on the services, and they receive unlimited care from the doctor, including unlimited cell phone calls any time of day or night. I think that's a little extreme, and for me there was an ethical conflict in asking people to pay up front for services they don't know they're ever going to receive. Unfortunately, I feel an ethical conflict in that some people can't afford to do what I'm doing. But I also see that I don't have a multitude of options – if I just worked with the insurance companies, I'd be back to the old game where I'd be in a hole. Now I work six sessions in my office a week – a session being a half-day – and I spend one afternoon a week at an eating disorders residential center, where I oversee the medical care. I can be at home the rest of the time. I carry my beeper, and I'm available for emergencies on days I'm not in the office, and half of the evenings and weekends.

I've found my lifestyle is acceptable now. I have enough time with my kids, and when I am on call, I no longer get dozens and dozens of phone calls because my patients are getting their needs met in the office. During the day, if they need a prescription they'll get the receptionist on the line; she'll take down their information; and the nurse will call in the prescription within an hour. It's going to happen, so they don't have to call me at eight o'clock in the evening and say, "My prescription was never filled." I also won't hear, "I was sick, but I couldn't get through on the phone," or "I knew I wouldn't get an appointment, so I didn't even bother calling."

I rarely get calls that aren't necessary. My patients don't want to call me on Saturday because they know I'm a person and that I'm out doing what I do. That's the whole point: *We are people to each other.* It's not me providing a service and them being pushed through the system. My kids are happier; they feel I'm more accessible. If they have to reach me during the day, they can page me, and I can take the five minutes between patients to call them back without getting backed up.

I feel blessed to have a career I enjoy. Of course there are pressures, and there are still days when I'm very stressed, but for the most part I feel my life is balanced, and I'm able to take care of myself. I don't have to wait 10 hours to go to the bathroom anymore! That's how I define success, for me. And I think my patients are happy.

Staying on Top of the Game

I like to use the technology available to keep up with my field. The Internet is wonderful for getting information; I can do MedLine searches from my home computer. The convenience is extraordinary. I don't have to pick up the *Physicians' Desk Reference;* I can just push a button now and get all the information I need about drugs. I listen to the drug company representatives when they come in – with a grain of salt, of course – because I have to know what new drugs are out, and by the time I get peer-reviewed medical information, some of these drugs have been out for a while, and my patients may have already started taking them. I have to keep up with the news media because patients often find things out before we do.

I have to go to continuing medical education courses to keep my accreditation, but I also go for myself, because I want to know what's happening. Recently I had to take board recertification. The American Board of Internal Medicine has required that physicians who took the exam in 1989 or later recertify 10 years later, so last year I went through a very long process, reviewing all the different topics in medicine. I had to complete take-home test modules; they give you three months to complete each one. That involved a lot of review and rereading. Then I had to study for a daylong sit-down test, which reminded me of my first set of boards. Anything I had missed, I picked up for that test.

I don't think board recertification was a waste of time, but I was not impressed with the way it was administered. It was not a good educational process. I think that rather than cramming everything into a year of studying for recertification, it should be an ongoing, continuing process, and there should be requirements for everyone to keep up. Right now a lot of people are "grandfathered" in and will never have to take the test. I do not think that will ever change, but I think we could use this as an ongoing process to self-evaluate, as well as for the board to evaluate us. Recertification does not need to be done all in one short period of time. Ten years after most people certify for the first time is usually a time when they are at a crucial period in their lives, in terms of families. Most of us have children, or we may be doing a lot of other things, and it's also a big career-building time. For me, it was especially difficult because I was caring for an elderly parent. I was really sandwiched and pushed during that year; I felt a lot of pressure. Fortunately, I deal fairly well under pressure, but I think people who don't would benefit from having board recertification stretched over a longer period.

I think it's important to set long-term goals, but I'm not a person for setting very picky, specific goals. I ask myself, "Do I want to be working more? Do I want to be working less? Do I want to know more about specific things?" When I started working with many patients with mind-body problems, I said, "In theory, I really like this work, and I have a lot of ideas about it, but I need better background." I was a psychology major in college, but that's a pretty vague background. So I looked around for ways I could learn more about theory and about psychobiology and psychopharmacology. A psychiatrist at the Philadelphia Association for Psychoanalysis (an organization mainly for psychologists, psychiatrists, and other therapists who are learning analysis) who was very interested in the border between psychiatry and medicine – mind and body – had started a fellowship that was free to non-psychiatrists with good ideas about what they would like to learn about the mind. He had been one of my teachers when I was a medical student rotating through psychiatry, and a friend reintroduced us. He encouraged my participation, so I took some courses there in the evenings, and did a lot of reading under the supervision of several of the senior psychiatrists. I undertook this with a lot of thought about how the information fit into my practice. Now I also look for conferences on mind-body medicine and psychopharmacology.

Once I think about what I want to know or what I want to learn, I will go out and look for ways to do it. I think planning for five years ahead, in terms of structural issues in the practice, is extremely important, as well. We look over our finances, the physical structure of the office, and the structure of how the staff is working. We ask ourselves what we need to have happen, so that a year from now things will be running just as smoothly, and a few new things can be implemented. For instance, right now we are considering a new database, and possibly having a gynecologist part-time in our space. Then we ask what will need to happen for us to still be running smoothly and have some loftier goals accomplished in five years – perhaps electronic medical records, for example. I think planning is important, but it's more of a gestalt than it is writing down goals one, two, and three. Also, circumstances and aspirations are always changing, and goals have to be reassessed frequently.

The Challenges of Being a Doctor

There are times when the responsibility of being a doctor feels overwhelming. It is particularly difficult when you have a patient who's not doing well and you cannot figure out what is wrong or what to do to make it better. In these situations it is important to know that you don't know. I used to always say, "Oh, I should be able to figure this out," but, in fact, none of us knows everything, and even if you know everything, sometimes you're too close to a situation – sometimes you look at the details, but can't see the whole picture. I will always call colleagues, sometimes specialists, because my patients often need a specialist who knows the finer points of certain diagnoses. Sometimes I need only to consult my partner, or another internist colleague. It's important to get past being ashamed of not knowing, and that was something that, unfortunately, we all carried with us from training. On rounds as a resident, if you were asked a question and didn't know the answer, it was an embarrassment. The fact is that many times you don't know, and you have to be able to say, "I really don't know what the situation is. I don't even know how to evaluate the next step. What do you think?"

I can't say there is a single person or type of person I would particularly like to emulate, but what I strive to be is a doctor who is always open to hearing what other people have to say – whether it's my patient, my staff, or other doctors. I strive to not be defensive and to not worry about my image too much because that impedes learning. I strive to emulate doctors who are humble, open, and honest. I don't try to emulate those doctors who have to say, "Oh, I knew that!" or, "Well, I think what I did was just as good!"

Another challenge I face is when something goes wrong in the doctor-patient relationship, and the communication isn't working right, and I wonder whether there was a better way to serve the patient. I think for me that's the hardest. I'm pretty self-critical, and I think about those things a lot. I think the best way to communicate with patients is face-to-face, always. I schedule regular follow-up visits with any patient who has complicated problems going on; it's very important to have regular visits set up. I've found that if we don't set up the regular visits, and there's a lot going on, and they don't show up again for three months, things will really start to fall apart for them. If they are coming to regular visits, they tend to pull it together; there's some accountability to me in face-to-face visits. We use the phone a lot in between visits, for questions and to communicate information back and forth (to discuss lab values or to talk about their visits with a consultant, for example). We use e-mail, although I don't like to. I've always been very resistant to technology; I was probably the last doctor on earth to get a cell phone, but once I got used to it, I got to the point where I couldn't do without it. I don't mind if patients e-mail me with simple questions or with requests for information; I just discourage them from using it to put a lot of their private information forward, because I think there are privacy issues. I also think that when you can't hear the person's tone of voice or see the other person's eyes, a lot of miscommunication can happen.

I would say that for most physicians, the time and financial pressure are now the hardest challenges to deal with. I feel lucky to not be quite so pressured with that. It's an overwhelming responsibility, and it's hard when I can't leave work in the office, and I bring it home with me in my head. Sometimes I think it would be nice to be doing something that would allow me to just walk out of my office and never think about work for a weekend, but that doesn't happen. When I go on vacation I call the office – not because I think they can't do without me, but because I want to know how somebody is doing, or I want to know how something turned out.

One of the largest current issues is malpractice. Malpractice insurance is prohibitively expensive for some of the subspecialists – physicians who do invasive surgery, particularly. Lawmakers have to handle that issue, unfortunately. In the Philadelphia area, one of the things that are driving the price of malpractice insurance up is litigation that has yielded a lot of large awards to patients with malpractice claims. Malpractice insurers feel this is a very risky area, so they've pulled out, or they're refusing to insure more doctors. In some cases insurance has become so expensive that some doctors can't afford to buy it and practice. We can't practice without malpractice insurance, so it puts everyone in a terrible bind.

I think the only solution for this problem is tort reform. There must be some limit on what people can sue for and how drawn-out these malpractice events will be. There may need to be some limits on awards, so that the malpractice insurers can actually insure people. In other countries with nationalized medicine, there are certainly malpractice suits, but not as many frivolous ones. I certainly would never want to see a patient who was harmed by true malpractice not receive what is due him or her. I often see a lot of "dragging the net," where a patient is harmed, and they or their attorneys may feel they have to file suit against not just the person who actually caused the problem, but also the drug company or the entire practice. So they drag the net and sue more people, and a lot of doctors then get involved in a lawsuit. These suits get drawn out for years, developing huge attorney fees and lost time. Those kinds of things drain the physicians emotionally and drain the financial system. Until we reform that process, we're going to have a malpractice crisis. If you look at what's going on in politics, you can see attempts to start reforming the process, but it will take a long time.

Figuring It All Out

I wish I could say I've received good advice, but I never had anybody to help me with that. I figured it out on my own – it was pretty rocky at times – and some of the things that happened to me along the way were less than ideal. One thing that happened that I think is important to point out is that I went through a serious illness myself. Fortunately, I ended up okay, but being a patient really showed me a lot about the whole world of medicine from the patient's point of view. It also taught me a great deal about striking a balance – that you just can't keep pushing yourself, and that eventually you will break down if you do that. So I guess much of the knowledge I eventually got was through trial by fire. I hope that as we see what is happening in medicine right now – the malpractice crises, the patient insurance crises, and the unhappy doctor crises – we'll learn we need to be teaching our future doctors more about striking the balance.

Learning the science of medicine comes primarily from schooling and training. It's important to go to a solidly good school, where you know you have top people in the field who are interested in teaching. One of the real crises right now is finding good academic physicians. Some medical schools have senior physicians who are so pressed to do their clinical work or research that teaching – which is never well compensated – falls by the wayside. It's important for young people interested in medicine to make sure they will interact with people who truly want to teach medical students, who truly want to instruct residents. Beyond that, learning the profession requires finding people to work with whose work you think is good, whom you admire, and whom you can ask for advice and emulate. I think it's very important to have mentors. I never had a mentor, but I always wished for one. Now I think I've found mentors – not one person who does everything ideally, but a variety of people. I work with so many psychiatric problems that I seek advice from psychiatrists and psychotherapists whose work I admire. My therapist colleagues can often help me sort out the psychological from the physiological. I also ask my partner, whom I trust very much, for help. I can review an unexpected situation with her, asking, "What do you think of what happened here?" and get good feedback. She always has up-to-the-minute drug information at her fingertips, and she approaches complicated problems in a thoughtful and systematic way. My husband, who is an academic internist and does a lot of teaching, is very helpful. He always knows where to find information and is very good with technology. I've learned from him. He also has always been a good role model with patient interaction – one of his areas of interest is teaching good patient interaction to medical students – so I trust his advice in dealing with difficult interactions. It's important to have a variety of people around you who have different talents you can draw on.

Since I changed my career path, I get calls from other doctors who are unhappy and are looking for other ways to practice medicine, and I hope I give some good advice. My favorite piece of advice to give other people is about self-care for doctors, particularly younger people who are in training now and trying to decide their future in medicine. I always say you have to take care of yourself first; you have to find a way to get sleep, eat reasonably, and exercise; and you have to be able to take care of your emotional needs. If you don't do that, you can't answer to patients as well.

These recent phone calls from other doctors saying, "How did you do this, and what do you think I should do?" have in some ways put me in a leadership position. If you want to be a leader in medicine, I think you have to take chances – never with patients, but with your office and the model of care you provide. A leader cannot be too focused on security – financial security or job security – because if that's what you're focused on, you're not going to be able to think about what it is that you really want in your career. It sounds a little bit hokey, but I think that if people would listen to their hearts and ask themselves, "What do I want to be?" and "What do I want to provide to my patients?" they would be much more successful. If you answer those questions and come up with a plan, the patients will come. If there are good doctors out there, patients will find them. Patients are desperate for good care. You shouldn't feel you have to stay in the system or that you have to practice medicine the way the majority of people are doing it. Concerns about job security will prevent you from finding a good way to practice medicine for yourself.

Stay Open to Future Changes

I think something big is going to happen in the world of financing medicine. I really don't know what it will be. I don't think our country is headed for socialized or nationalized medicine because of the very capitalist interest of the country, and I don't think the big-money people will let that happen. But something will happen. I've seen too many doctors leave my area because they cannot afford their malpractice insurance, or leave medicine because they're so unhappy. I don't know exactly how these issues will resolve themselves. I think some of it might swing back to what I'm doing – the "old-fashioned way," like when I was a kid and you used to go to the doctor, pay the doctor, and if you had medical insurance you submitted the claim and got back what you got. I think that will be at least part of what will happen – that more and more doctors will start practicing the way I do, or in some similar form.

In the future I hope patients and doctors will come to more of an understanding of each other's position. Patients want and need a lot of things from their physicians, and right now physicians' hands are pretty tied. The reason people are angry at some physicians and at the way the world of medicine is working is that they're not getting their needs met. I hope we will eventually meet in the middle to gain an understanding of each other and find a way to work things out.

To prepare for these changes I think it's very important to be forward-thinking and flexible. In the time I've been practicing medicine things have changed drastically. I have to understand that they're going to continue to change, and that I may have to change my plans. If we did go into a nationalized system, my whole practice would have to change, and I think I have to be open to that. You have to say, "OK, whatever will happen will happen, but I still want to practice medicine, and I will still have to look for my niche and my place." I think one of the sad things that happened to the older physicians is that they didn't foresee the system of HMOs coming. When it hit, their practices were so altered, and they were disappointed and disillusioned. They had worked so hard, and now all of a sudden they were told they had to practice a radically different way. We have to be looking ahead all the time. Change will happen, and we have to be open to it.

Seeing the Human Being

A lot of people think the only physician's oath is the Hippocratic Oath. The Hippocratic Oath is certainly important, in that it basically says we'll practice our art and science ethically. But the other physician's oath is the Oath of Maimonides, which says, "Inspire me with love for my art and for your creatures; in the sufferer let me only see the human being."

I would say that if there's one rule for being a physician, it's seeing the human being in the patient. If you do that, it forces you both to practice ethically and to do your best. I think we also have to stay humble; practicing medicine is a humbling experience, and we will all make mistakes. Talking about our mistakes has been terribly discouraged in the medical world for as long as I can remember. The concern about malpractice is one reason not to talk about mistakes, but the other reason is the shame that you didn't know or you didn't do something right. We need to be humble, realizing that we all make mistakes, that there's always a time when someone else could have done it better, and that there's always another way that it could have been done. If you allow yourself to know that you can learn, and then you'll really be working in the best interest of the patient.

Dr. Rosalind Kaplan is a board-certified internist in private practice in Haverford, Pennsylvania. She earned her M.D. degree at the University of Pennsylvania School of Medicine and completed post-graduate training at Temple University Hospital in Philadelphia. She also completed a two-year clinical fellowship with the Philadelphia Association for Psychoanalysis, studying psychosomatics.

After several years in academic medicine, Dr. Kaplan began in private practice, treating general medical problems, as well as the medical complications of eating disorders. She serves as a medical consultant to the Renfrew Center, a residential facility for eating disorders.

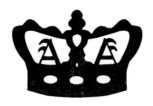

WHAT IS A "GOOD DOCTOR"?

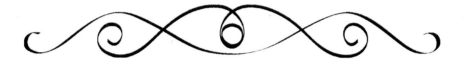

MARIANNE J. LEGATO, M.D.
Columbia University College of Physicians & Surgeons

Partnership for Gender-Specific Medicine
Founder and Director

The Personal Difference

As she was driving me to my medical school graduation, my mother said something to me that has informed my whole career. She said, "I just want you to know that you can't be a good doctor without being a good person." I remember feeling skeptical at the time: I thought that simply mastering a critical mass of important knowledge would guarantee I'd be successful. But I never forgot what she said, and I now think it was the most provocative piece of advice I've ever been given. Through my vocation, I've learned to control my temper and my demand for immediate results. I've learned the importance of patience and of being completely truthful. I've learned not to take advantage of people who are weak and compromised. I truly believe that if I have developed at all as a human being, a lot of it has to do with the demands of my particular profession, which requires a high standard of personal virtue. *probably true.*

There are no perfect doctors; there are only "good enough" doctors. Good doctors are dedicated to the welfare of their patients and try never to harm or exploit them. Good doctors, in general, admit when they don't know the answers to questions. Good doctors have a good enough critical mass of up-to-date knowledge and information that if people are ill (or think they're ill), their doctors can effectively help them. But simply knowing a lot of facts isn't enough: A really effective doctor must be a well-integrated, mature, empathetic, and courteous individual. Regard and respect for patients is an essential ingredient of effective treatment. Cultural, social, and economic information about the patient is important to understanding how best to help them. That's why house calls aren't a burden, but a wonderful chance to add essential elements to what we know about the patient and how to marshal the best resources to cure or palliate his illness. In short, personal qualities make the difference between a good doctor and a great doctor.

There are a few giants in medicine: Soma Weiss, the famous Harvard physician, or Robert Loeb, one of the greatest of the physicians who taught at Columbia's College of Physicians & Surgeons, are two fine examples. Those men seemed to know everything about illness, and they were impeccably gifted at diagnosis. While I remember them as great scholars, the doctors I most admire not only have state-of-the-art information about their subspecialty, but they are also always available for advice and consultation. They don't send the house staff or their junior partners to care for problems because it's late at night or a Sunday; they come themselves. They accept personal, consistent, and complete responsibility for their patients.

On the day I graduated from medical school, my mother gave me a copy of the Hippocratic Oath, which one of her own mentors had given to her. I still read it at least once a week and think about what an important promise it is and how it embodies a tremendously important series of principles on which to build a professional life. The Oath reminds me that our vocation is unique: We are privy to the innermost thoughts of patients; we are a screen on which they paint their most terrible fears, their hopes, and their interpretation of the world around them. Doctors have to remain the custodians and the guardians of that information; we must not talk about what we learn in the course of our lives with patients, nor ever exploit them in any way, even when they will never find out about it. Some people have called this profession a form of priesthood, and I think that's not too strong a word; we do perform a unique service.

yeah – I guess you have to think you're superman

One of the most important parts of growing to be an ever more effective doctor is to try to perfect personal virtue. It is important to be truthful, courageous, and persistent and not to surrender to fear in the face of such terrible realities as illness, decay, and death. The doctor must learn to accept that some patients will die and be prepared to help them deal with that. That means keeping them company during that time, not turning away from them and leaving them alone when nothing more can be done to lessen the impact of the illness or to save their lives.

some?

Successful physicians have to set realistic goals. You can't cure all people; you can't cure all illness; and you can't stop all pain, discomfort, and anxiety. Accepting that and not taking it personally when a patient becomes enraged if you don't do those things is also part of being a successful physician. Another good measure of success is how often your colleagues call you for advice or consultation – whether it's formal or informal. In a competitive and often professionally jealous world, it's reassuring if good doctors ask your opinion on complex issues.

Hmm

The Doctor-Patient Relationship

For me, the best part of being a doctor is the relationship with the individual patient. That partnership is the essence of medical practice. Part of its success depends on courteous and empathetic attention to the patient, an ability to support the patient in times of difficulty, and the ability to offer reassurance and be a resource for the patient. The relationship is not between equals, in the sense that the patient, as a famous psychoanalyst once explained to me, is sick, regressed, and vulnerable. In my experience it requires daily vigilance to control such inappropriate responses to patients as unwarranted anger, frustration, and irritation.

In approaching the doctor-patient relationship, a few principles are very helpful. First, not every patient is for every doctor, and the first interview is a careful assessment of whether or not you are an appropriate match for the patient, and whether or not you can be helpful – two different things. Having the courage to say, after a sophisticated assessment, "I cannot help you" – which I've done in my own practice – is an important thing to know how to do.

Second, don't abandon your patient if the patient can't collaborate in carrying out what you think is the best treatment for him. For example, a patient may have weighed over 300 pounds for most of his adult life. While you can explain that it would be very important to lose 100 of those pounds, he may simply not be able to accomplish that. It becomes really important to explain, then, that this is something you can work on together, but that you won't abandon him if he in fact can't successfully lose weight. Supporting the patient according to his ability to carry out your recommendations, not according to what he "should" do, is very important.

Third, you must keep in touch with the patient, even when the patient is disaffected or angry or frightened. If the patient is unpleasant or difficult, it's reasonable to ask, "Why are you so upset?" at least a few times, and to try to get close to the problem rather than ignore it. If a patient turns out to be inconsolable, you can then say, "Perhaps I can help you find another doctor who might be more helpful to you, because I believe you need care."

wiser

A patient's unrealistic expectations are a significant challenge for a doctor. Patients would like you to be a magical individual – able to cure all their pain and to rescue them from their illness, no matter how terrible it is. They may ask you for inappropriate things: to be their parent instead of their physician, or even to be a magician. More than one patient has said to me at the end of a long recital of terrible complaints, "Now I want you to wave a magic wand and make all of this go away." Sometimes the patient has an inappropriate response to the physician – they want to make the doctor a personal friend or even a romantic object. Your responsibility as the more powerful, idealized person in the relationship is to gently turn away these inappropriate impulses.

No!
Who?

About 2 percent of cases are terribly concerning. They are a combination of a very sick patient and no diagnosis. When I encounter this, my first reaction is to involve the best brains I can to help me, and we literally discuss the patient several times a day. It's very important to keep the patient in the loop as new ideas for diagnosis and treatment develop: to tell the patient what's going on, to let him know how much communication is going on about him, and to explain – either on the phone or in person – exactly what we're thinking. Keeping the flow of information to the patient constant is crucial, so that even if we don't have an answer, the patient doesn't feel abandoned or terrified.

Learning to listen to the patient without letting your mind wander is an important skill to cultivate. It requires you to shut out all distracting thoughts and outside intrusions during the interview. Control of the interview is also critical. I have patients who will digress so much that they eat up the time that's allotted before you can get the facts you need to be most effective. Often this happens because the patient is too frightened to be direct: They resist telling me what's really bothering them.

Controlling the flow of information so that you have the data you need without offending or cutting off the patient requires you to use your senses of smell, sight, touch, and hearing. Sometimes the signals are right before our eyes. I watch the color of the skin of my patient as he tells me his story. Some patients come in gray with anxiety, and it's only when the color begins to return to their faces that I understand that they are less frightened and more at ease.

The doctor-patient relationship is not an equal relationship. A doctor is perceived as much more powerful – and *is,* by virtue of his or her knowledge and ability to intervene. As much as modern society likes to say the patient should take charge, the patient can't; the patient doesn't have the training, the objectivity, or the freedom from personal terror to take charge of his or her own case.

Doctors must be careful to remember the vulnerability of the patient and not exploit it. Sometimes patients want to please you; they think that by being "good patients," they'll get better results from you. Sometimes they have skills or access to things that would be helpful to you, and you must never ask them for that without thinking very carefully about it. If you're writing a book, for example, and your patient is a famous publisher, it's hard to resist asking the patient for help. That may not be appropriate if the patient is ill, and you should never approach them about such things in the consulting room. That place and that time is exclusively for them and should never be contaminated with your irrelevant personal needs or demands.

No! Who?

wow! You mean doctors have those?

Working With the Staff

An office "staff" – whether it's one person or 40 people – is terribly important to a successful practice. After all, your patient's first experience with you is actually through contact with others: It's others who make the appointment, others who explain to the patient what he should expect when he makes his first visit to the office. A good office nurse can be very consoling and reassuring to a patient. On the other hand, I think it's very important not to let your staff members overstep their responsibilities by interpreting tests or giving the patient information that is best left to the physician to explain.

Respect for staff is as essential as respect for the patient. Bursts of short temper and rudeness or even underpaying them will undermine their ability to function. They are partners in patient care and should be treated as such. Personal qualities of humor and an ability to take very disparate and often very entrepreneurial individuals and meld them into a team are crucial. A doctor who can collaborate and not dictate, but also lead others to achieve important and mutually acceptable goals, will be an effective practitioner.

The Medical Profession: Past, Present, and Future

Before World War II, we couldn't do much to intervene in the course of illness. We had no antibiotics; anesthesia was not very sophisticated; and our art was better developed than our science. We were experts at keeping patients company and paid exquisite attention to every detail of the patient's illness. We described it and predicted what would happen; our entire attention was devoted to the sick person.

After WWII the burst of important science that was developed – in medicine, but also in the broader world of scientific technology – refocused our attention on the phenomenon of "testing" the patient. Through the combination of an abundance of technology and its apparent power in an increasingly litigious environment, we came to feel that it's better to have the results of a "test," which is a black-and-white matter, than the details of a patient's account of his illness. A "test" was positive or negative, reliable, and provided a better defense if we were criticized. As a group we began to retreat from the bedside of the patient, into the chart and the data. We found ourselves literally making rounds at a table with a patient's charts, and losing our ability – if we ever had it, depending on our age – to really see, hear, and examine the patient and to relate primarily to him or her. We became "dataphiles," and our fascination with technology and the black-and-white nature of the laboratory chart has reinforced a turning away from the patient.

My personal aim – one of them – as a faculty member at a major institution is to reacquaint the medical students and the trainees, and even my own colleagues, with the story of the patient's illness, as told by the patient. I think the patient is ultimately the best teacher; he or she asks some of the best questions and gives us some of the most accurate information about the experience of illness, its symptoms, and the details of its course. I also think that, for me – although I like data as much as the next person – the richest part of being a physician is that interchange with the patients. I find the patient is the true point of the exercise and the most fascinating of its aspects.

I now give a lecture to students on the art and science of physical diagnosis before they have their first real contact with the sick. When we go on rounds, I like to leave the chart far behind and go to the bedside to teach people how to learn about illness directly from the patient. I don't think managed care or a third-party payer has caused our increasing distance from the sick person; I think technology has caused this tremendous change in focus and emphasis. *interesting*

A major concern of mine for the future of medicine is the problem of malpractice suits. I think what's happened to physicians is rather shocking. We live in a litigious society, and I think doctors are inadequately protected from malpractice suits. Insurance premiums have rocketed skyward, consuming a significant portion of practice income. Simply being accused of malpractice can be crippling: I think the public believes that if you're sued, you're not as good a doctor as if you're not sued. More and more people are leaving medicine because of the malpractice costs and the risk of a suit. Doctors do not set out to do harm, and, I think, contrary to public opinion, we do an excellent job of policing one another. I don't know any other profession that is as certified and recertified as ours, or whose ongoing training and scrutiny is as intense as our own.

My particular interest in medicine is in exploring and explaining the reasons for the differences between the normal function of men and women and in the differences in how they experience disease. We call the new science gender-specific medicine, and I believe it will inform the way we practice medicine in the future. I think as we learn more, we understand much more fully that men and women are not identical. We are correcting what I call the "bikini view" of women – that breast health and reproductive biology are the only important areas that are different between the two sexes. In fact, women are not small men, and we can't restrict our research to male subjects as we have done in the past.

Also, I'm confident there will be a return to interest in the patient. I think the public will demand and reward that in physicians. And I believe that if we intend to keep the best and the brightest people in medicine, we're going to start rewarding them for their efforts, both financially and in protecting them from malpractice suits that have little or no basis for existing.

Dr. Marianne J. Legato is an internationally known academic physician, author, lecturer, and specialist in women's health. She is a professor of Clinical Medicine at Columbia University College of Physicians & Surgeons and the founder and director of the Partnership for Gender-Specific Medicine at Columbia University. She is a practicing internist in New York City.

Dr. Legato has spent her research career on cardiovascular research on the structure and function of the cardiac cell. The American Heart Association and the National Institutes of Health supported her work. She won the Murray Steele Award, the Martha Lyon Slater Fellowship, and a four-year Senior Investigator Award from the American Heart Association, New York Affiliate. She won a coveted Research Career Development Award from the National Institutes of Health and sat on the National Heart Lung and Blood Institute's study section on cardiovascular disease, as well as the Basic Science Council of the American Heart Association. Most recently, she has served as a charter member of the Advisory Board of the Office of Research on Women's Health of the National Institutes of Health, and she received the "Woman in Science" award from the American Medical Women's Association in February 2002.

In 1992 Dr. Legato won the American Heart Association's Blakeslee Award for the best book written for the lay public on cardiovascular disease with her publication of The Female Heart: The Truth About Women and Heart Disease. Her newest book for the lay public on gender-specific medicine, Eve's Rib, was published in spring 2002.

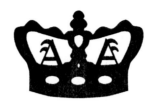

THE INCREDIBLE VALUE OF BEING WITH YOUR PATIENTS

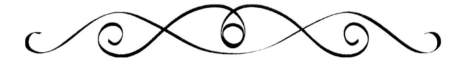

MARC BORENSTEIN, M.D.
Newark Beth Israel Medical Center

Department of Emergency Medicine
Chairman and Residency Director

133

The Need for the Warm and Fuzzy

My lifelong career in medicine and my professional mission have been dedicated to the incorporation of humanistic values and the art of medicine into the clinical knowledge base and scientific technology that form the foundation for all physicians independent of their chosen specialty. For many years the art of medicine was not formally taught. Rather, it was observed and learned at the side of a mentor with the hope that somehow it would filter through to the student through a process of osmosis. Some elements of the art of medicine, such as the ability to form relationships with people, the ability to communicate, and the demonstration of empathy, were thought to be in the realm of "soft" science, often referred to as "warm and fuzzy stuff." It was generally thought that these areas could not be readily taught, nor was credible research possible, since these areas were not subject to the rigor and scientific discipline that could be applied to disciplines such as biochemistry, physiology, and scientific technology.

Medical training involves the mastery of a substantial knowledge base, which starts in high school and college. It requires training and education in a variety of basic chemical and biological sciences. In medical school students spend approximately two years studying the clinical sciences, such as anatomy, physiology, embryology, pharmacology, and biochemistry, and then another two years understanding the application of these sciences to specific medical disciplines and clinical care, thereby learning the basic approach to the major medical specialties. Clinical rotations of varying duration in medical specialties, such as pediatrics, internal medicine, surgery, obstetrics and gynecology, and psychiatry, are usually required in medical school curricula. Additional clinical rotations in such disciplines as radiology, the surgical subspecialties (urology, ophthalmology, plastic surgery, otorhinolaryngology), and emergency medicine may be required in some medical schools or taken on an elective basis in others.

As students progress through their medical education and subsequent residency training, they acquire many technical and procedural skills. These range from basic procedures mastered in medical school, such as starting an intravenous line, drawing blood samples, and inserting a bladder catheter, to the highly advanced and invasive procedures, requiring many months to years of training, such as surgical endoscopy, heart and major blood vessel catheterizations, and surgical operations. Acquisition and mastery of these skills and scientific knowledge are daunting. Despite the long and highly publicized hours of residency, it soon becomes apparent to the medical novice, often referred to as an intern, that there is insufficient time to do everything that must get done and to learn everything that must be learned.

Most interns and residents are overwhelmed with the enormous demands placed upon them to just get the tasks and documentation done that are required for delivering correct and complete medical care in a hospital. Every day (and night) is filled with obtaining and writing medical histories, performing physical examinations, ordering and checking laboratory tests and diagnostic imaging studies, studying about uncommon medical conditions, reading medical journals, going on rounds with faculty and attending physicians, and, whenever and wherever possible, getting sleep. As a result these highly motivated but forever busy house officers pay little attention to acquiring skills in such areas as communication, conflict resolution, bringing out the best in others, and building relationships. Experiencing the emotional content of medicine and getting in touch with one's own emotions occurring during the intimacy of delivering medical care are not only irrelevant to completing the tasks of medicine, but can actually be perceived as obstructive to the rapid, efficient completion of these tasks. As residency progresses, many physicians in training not only lose touch with the humanistic elements of medicine, but some have it actively driven out of them through role modeling that covertly, or even overtly, communicates that it is detrimental or weak to have any emotional connection to the patient.

Ironically, during the past 50 to 60 years, as teaching in humanism and the art of medicine was decreasing in formal medical education and residency training, public yearning for a return to humanism and the art of medicine increased. As we began to approach the end of the 20th century, an increasing public awareness that humanism is essential to the role of physicians as healers and to the role of medicine as a healing science became evident. During this time, as we have become more and more scientifically advanced, people are yearning for connections to each other and themselves on a more soulful and spiritual basis. It is probably no coincidence that with the tremendous technological advances over the past 60 years in medical science, there have been new and very popular movements to preserve the humanistic elements in medicine. For example, look at the alternative medicine movement that is now a major aspect of healthcare delivery in our country. It would not be surprising to find that the majority of people in the United States have some type of alternate care. Practices such as herbal therapy, acupuncture, and massage therapy, which might have appeared unusual in 1973, are now commonplace. Herbal remedies, such as Echinacea, St. John's wort, and saw palmetto, are mass produced today and sold in supermarkets alongside vitamins, aspirin, and acetaminophen. In addition, you see that people today want and need to participate in not only how their healthcare is delivered, but also in how their babies are actually delivered into the world, as well as how they leave the world in old age.

It is interesting that if you look at post-WWII America in, say, the 1950s, it is apparent that we entered the scientific convenience era characterized by a widespread availability of everything from frozen food, television, and refrigerators, to automatic transmissions. During this time, hospitals became very prominent as centers for medical care where people went for everything from birth to death. Along with this development of the hospital as the center for medical care was a paternalistic culture in medicine in which doctors said, "We know what is best for you, and we will tell you what needs to be done." At the 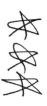 height of this era, a great birthing experience was viewed as something along the lines of a woman being knocked out with light anesthesia toward the end of her labor. Subsequently, she was found waking up with her baby, all clean and tidy, being placed in her arms by a nurse, thereby missing the whole birthing experience with a painless and unconscious process. During the entire time of labor, fathers were sent away, to be summoned back by the physician at some point after the baby was born. From that extreme scenario, we have seen a continued demand for the conscious, active participation of both the mother and the father in the birthing process. There has been a dramatic rise in requests for natural childbirth, fathers at the bedside throughout labor, Lamaze methods, non-hospital birthing centers, and use of midwives.

You see the same thing with death. In the 19th century it was common for birth and death to take place in the house. Families living in one home were often multigenerational. Both children and adults were present to witness the process of birth and death. As hospitals, technology, and science in general moved forward in the 20th century, morbidity and mortality from labor and delivery for both mother and child decreased. Home delivery with its greater risks became unacceptable to obstetrical specialists. Pregnant women went to the hospital for birthing. Elderly people with serious illness were sent to the hospital where they died. A death in the household became unusual. In our times it is possible to meet someone 20 or 25 years old and discover they have never seen anybody die; this was not the case 100 years ago. Today the use of advance directives, living wills, and so on, indicate that people want clear participation and a say in how they die and to what extent advanced medical technology or resuscitative efforts are to be used in their medical treatment.

The human element and the art of medicine have become very important expectations for most people who want them to be part of their medical care. In his book *Megatrends,* John Nesbit called this phenomenon "high tech, high touch." That is, the greater the amount and sophistication of technology in medical care, the more people will be looking for some type of touch and feel – *HMM* they didn't want to be just a number in a complex technologic process; they wanted the human element to be preserved. Paying attention to people's individuality and interacting with them in a way that gives them the experience of being cared about as a person is very important to them.

When I look at the attention being placed on the art of medicine today, what is interesting to me is the increasing focus on how to teach it. In fact, the Accreditation Council for Graduate Medical Education over the past few years has developed, in association with the American Medical Association and others, something called the six core competencies, which are being incorporated into the training requirements for every specialty in medicine. Two of the core competencies have to do with professionalism, communication, and those qualities that one might call the art of medicine, such as humanism. These competencies have now been formalized and defined to a high degree, so they can be taught with more rigor than they have been in the past.

Necessary Qualities

Some of the necessary qualities for a physician that were referred to more than 100 years ago as the three A's were affability, availability, and ability. These still hold true today. Traditionally, the narrow definition of affability is likableness or pleasantness,

accessible? – you can get to me
available? – I can do it

but it goes beyond that in medicine. One needs what is broadly defined as professionalism, which includes the talent and ability to form relationships, acknowledge others generously, communicate, provide service, and demonstrate empathy, care, and concern for others. Availability is certainly essential. If one does not have access to healthcare, especially for emergency medical care, from a regional or national perspective or to the doctor on an individual basis in the doctor-patient relationship, then things break down. Ability is basically everything it takes to do the job right.

It is essential for the physician to experience a sense of calling to the profession. Medicine is not for everyone. It requires that you place the welfare of others before your own personal desires and needs. That is what drives physicians to put in the hours that they put in during residency or to do whatever it takes to get the job done. I believe that is what drives the physician to not only be awake while on duty all night but to be alert and even hypervigilant. That driver is a mandate that comes from within. It is experienced as innate and fundamental. It is a quality of being that calls you to put the needs of others before your own, to have an innate desire to be of service to others and to enhance the quality of life through greater well-being and health for people. That does not mean you cannot be compensated for your work or have other interests in life, such as traveling or enjoying leisure activities. At the same time, if you were to enter medicine only for personal gain, such as social prestige or financial compensation or other self-centered reasons, the inner sense of motivation and innate drive would simply not be great enough to pull you through when the going gets tough. Ironically, you might still be able to deliver great technical care, and patients might be all the better for it, but an inner sense of fulfillment and satisfaction would in all likelihood be missing both for the physician and the patient. So you have to have the sense that this is a calling and that it's your life's work. I don't think this is, however, unique to medicine and the healthcare profession. People in professions as diverse as theater, art, music, teaching, and other social and community services, such as firefighters and police officers, have that similar sense of placing community service and contribution to society above one's personal needs and desires.

[handwritten margin notes: "FINALLY!", "Someone realized that!"]

Certainly a physician must also have intellectual ability and a substantial amount of specialized knowledge. But perhaps more important, there must be a view of study as an ongoing journey – a willingness to stay fresh and current, to abandon certain ideas and viewpoints when newer perspectives render a particular mode of thinking obsolete. There is an old phrase called "hardening of the attitudes," which has been said in medicine to be worse than hardening of the arteries. If you have that condition in medicine, you will be especially unlikely to provide great care as you progress through your career. This is because attitudes and opinions in large part shape who we are with patients, and it is who we are that determines what patients will be left with as an experience of us.

Traditional medical education devotes substantial time to teaching physicians what to do. As a residency director, I am constantly asked by my residents what to do in every situation. I am frequently asked by my interns in emergency medicine, "If a patient comes in with a myocardial infarction, can you just tell me what I should do?" As they advance in residency, the quest for knowing what to do becomes more specific and detailed, "If a patient comes in with an inferior wall myocardial infarction complicated by hypotension and bradycardia, what do I do?" In addition to performing the tasks necessary for providing the correct medical treatment, residents also want to do medical procedures correctly, accurately. And we train them to perform the right medical tasks for providing medical treatments or performing medical procedures. However, little time, if any, is spent exploring who we are with patients when we are performing the right tasks. Patients have no way of evaluating if what I am doing as a physician is medically correct. They take for granted that I am placing the sutures in the right location and that the laceration even needs sutures. Patients usually do not even remember what I am doing. They will, however, remember with great clarity who I am while I was with them doing whatever I was doing.

The problem for the physician and people in general is that we are oblivious to who we are being with people. We have our attention on what we are doing. So if I am being quiet while I am placing the sutures (perhaps because in my world, being quiet is how I focus and concentrate), the patient may leave with an experience of me as being aloof, rude, or disinterested (perhaps because in the patient's world, quiet communicates dislike). This mismatch of experiences usually remains concealed to both the patient and the physician during the medical encounter but may surface in a patient satisfaction survey in which the patient writes, "The doctor was uninterested in me," and gives the doctor a poor rating. The doctor, in turn, receives this commentary and with great frustration states, "I did everything right for that patient, meticulously suturing a complex laceration, giving it far more attention for a great cosmetic closure than most physicians would have. What is the matter with that patient?" Thus, for a physician to be able to deliver excellent medical care (all the right things done right) and provide that medical care in a manner that makes the patient feel taken care of and valued as a person, it is essential for the physician to use external experiences of others as a mirror to gain insight into how he or she is with others that might not be apparent from an internal viewpoint of oneself. *Let others reflect you to you* *Everybody should do that.*

A physician must have an innate interest in how his or her behavior affects others and a desire to gain access into how his or her behavior is experienced by others. There used to be a time when much was overlooked with regard to the ability to form relationships, communicate, and provide people with an experience of being taken care of and valued as a person. Even today you hear people say, "That doctor has no bedside manner, but he is a great surgeon in the operating room." Some patients will say, "I don't care what his or her bedside manner is – I just want someone who can take my gall bladder out without any complications." But more and more we are seeing that it is not sufficient to have the technical skill without the human elements. Patients are increasingly unwilling to settle for half of what they want. The public wants it all. *DAMN PUBLIC!*

To be successful, today's physicians need their work to come from the heart. They need to love others and be moved by that *?*

concern for others. They need to have some type of burning desire to achieve excellence, to go on a life's journey of learning and teaching, and to retain the qualities of empathy and compassion. The word "demonstrate" must be used pointedly, because you cannot just feel something internally and expect others to see it. When you are working with people, it is essential that qualities such as empathy be demonstrated outwardly by who you are being so that others experience it.

As a doctor you have to listen. The power of listening is extraordinary, so listen to your patients and to others, and listen for new ideas and fresh approaches. Find the good in everybody. See the value in each person and what they contribute to the well-being of the patient. If you put patients first, almost everything else will become clear about what needs to be done in a given situation. Also, put the needs of others ahead of yourself and focus on the concept of service and its value as a contribution to the world.

The pursuit of knowledge and the willingness to continually grow as a person, and to teach and contribute to others, are important qualities in a physician. Notice that none of these things have to do with getting an "A" on your exams or doing well on the MCATs. We do look at those things when people apply to medical school and our residency, as it is important to have a command of our knowledge base, but a lot information can be looked up. It is surprising how much information can be looked up and how often information does not make the difference anyway, because in life it seems that we often know what to do but are just not doing it.

Of course, information is very important, but we often know where to get it. It is applying the behaviors and actions and interacting with people and the world in a way that makes the world a better place that is important – things that don't get measured on a test. In the end tests are not what make the difference. What counts is paying attention to detail, thinking that everything matters, and that every aspect of how you interact with a patient can contribute to their well-being.

No job in providing medical care is too small. For example, it has been shown that patients who feel someone in the healthcare profession cares about them as a person heal faster. They spend less time in a hospital and die less often. So, if a hospital transporter is taking a patient from on a 10-minute trip from the emergency department to a bed in the hospital and interacts with the patient in a way that the patient feels valued and cared for, then that transporter could actually contribute to that patient's well-being. The patient might actually heal faster and possibly even leave the hospital sooner. That is an amazing thought: that a hospital transporter might have something to do with decreasing patient's length of stay. We do not tend to think that way, nor do we think to examine the performance and contribution of excellence in the jobs such as hospital transporter. All too often, hospital management may overlook these types of jobs and the persons who have been hired for them, thinking that anyone can do the job. But excellence in any job is highly important and valuable. And excellence in hospital transport services may have the potential for far more impact in the hospital than just transport time from A to B. We do know that when people feel better about themselves as a person they heal better. So who is to say that the person transporting a patient could not make the difference in that patient feeling better about himself or herself as a person?

The Doctor as a Leader

The qualities and characteristics that contribute to effective leadership are not the same qualities and characteristics that are essential to being a great physician. Sometimes physicians find themselves in positions of management and leadership because of excellence in areas such as research and clinical care – excellence in these areas generates a great deal of respect in our profession, and thus it is possible to be elevated to a position of leadership or management as a result. However, such a physician may not necessarily have the skills to motivate others, because leadership requires an ability to articulate a vision and be in touch with a sense of purpose. To be a leader in medicine, you have to walk the walk and talk the talk. But it is essential that you do so as a natural expression of who you are.

Leadership requires that we bring out the best in others, and our accountability as leaders is measured by the productivity and outcomes that others produce. Many physicians are trained to produce outcomes by themselves. Often they are taught not to trust the work of others and to check everything personally. This healthy skepticism can have potentially life-saving benefits for patients. At the same time, these physicians may have a quality of the "lone ranger" and not work well with others or be effective in leading others. When you are trained to produce

146

outcomes yourself, that is different from working with others in such a way that your success is measured by the outcomes they produce. It is the difference between coaching and playing in a sport – some people can bridge that gap and are very successful at both; some people are great coaches but not great players; and some people are great players but not necessarily great coaches. So I think many times the necessary skill sets and what you are naturally called to do as a doctor are different from what is required to be a leader.

I have been a residency director or involved with building residency programs for about 14 years, and I actually see part of my life's mission as working with others to help them be their best, to fulfill their dreams, and to achieve things they did not think were possible. When people apply to my residency program, I tell them I am interested in people who want to work with people. I am interested in working with people who are looking to take on more in life than they thought might have been possible for them before they started residency training. There has to be some natural motivation to take these sorts of positions because they take more time and are more all-consuming, so it had better be something you love. You have to be enthusiastic and have a natural tendency toward optimism – you have to be able to make lemonade from lemons and take time to "mine for the gold" in people and in situations. You have to be able to keep people focused on their missions.

Mother Teresa once said:

> People are unreasonable, illogical, and self-centered. Love them anyway. If you do good,

You'll be scared. Do it anyway)

people will accuse you of selfish ulterior motives. Do good anyway. If you are successful, you will win false friends and true enemies. Succeed anyway. Honesty and frankness make you vulnerable. Be honest and frank anyway. People really need help but may attack you if you help them. Help them anyway. Give the world the best you have, and you will get kicked in the teeth. Give the world the best you have anyway.

I think you have to have some of that attitude as a physician.

Margaret Mead said, "Never doubt that a small group of committed citizens can change the world. Indeed it is the only thing that ever has." These are some of the ideas and philosophies regarding life that give me inspiration in seeking to deliver excellence in healthcare, no matter what. Today, especially in the emergency department where we provide care for so many people who might otherwise not have access to healthcare, our mission is to deliver excellence and create an environment where anybody can walk in and have an experience of dignity. My mission is to train people to be true to that. We have not gotten there yet, but it is worth working on.

The Importance of Being With and Communicating With Patients

As mentioned earlier, people are often aware of what they are doing, but they are not often aware of who they are *being* when they are doing it. Frequently we pay attention to training people in terms of what to do, but not how to be with people. For example, if I am starting an intravenous line, I may use all the necessary techniques to get the job done, but the patient may not feel taken care of. The patient's feeling taken care of is a function of who I am being with the patient. Am I being kind, caring, a good listener? These are all in the domain of *being*. It is a very interesting and important area, but we do not spend a lot of time on this in teaching.

Most of us are not aware of who we are being. But often the only thing patients remember is who we were being. They cannot actually assess the technical aspects of what we are doing. It is similar to the airline industry, which has been used as an analogy in patient satisfaction and service. When we look at airplane travel, we often use what are called surrogate indicators to determine what airline we will choose for travel. Surrogate indicators include things like the comfort of the seats or the pleasantness of the flight attendants. What really matters, though, is how often a particular airline services the airplane engines or how often they train pilots and update them on new technology or flight simulators. We do not tend to think about that; we just assume it's all done.

Similarly, when you walk into an emergency department, you assume the doctor knows what he or she is doing. We do not get any points for putting the stitches in the right place, and you would not even know if we put them in the right place, anyway, because you cannot really evaluate that. If, while I am suturing, I appear to be distant and uncommunicative, people will tend to personalize what is going on and may assume that my disposition has something to do with them. Most of us tend to take our past experiences and incorporate them into the present, so a patient might assume the doctor is not appearing friendly because the patient is on welfare, or because of his or her racial background. It may have nothing to do with that, and yet that is the conclusion they draw. So it is extremely important that we teach our physicians to be aware of who they are being with patients. It's also important to remember that a neutral way of being doesn't work, either, because people don't know how to interpret neutral. You have to actually *show* compassion with your voice, your facial expressions, and mannerisms.

A number of communication approaches or techniques can be taught, but none of them is a substitute for innate sincerity and a love for people. That can't be taught; it has to be there from the start. Unless you are in a removed research arena in which you have no contact with patients, medicine is a people specialty, where you work with people. No matter how you look at various equations and scientific processes, as soon as you inject the human element, it is people, and they do not conform to all the formulas; people are not algebra or geometry. It's important to appreciate that we are working with people, to have a basic love of people, and to learn from the people you come in contact with.

The old saying, "Physician, heal thyself," has to do with the notion that there is a personal journey available to a physician, and the access to that journey is through the patients and other people we work with and come in contact with, such as the nursing, healthcare, and management staff, and family and friends. Once you start with that, there are ways to open things up with patients.

When you first meet a patient, introduce yourself, and let the patient know who you are and what your role is in their healthcare. It sounds very basic, but it is so important. If the patient has been referred to you in your office, that relationship may already be there. In emergency medicine, however, the vast majority of people we encounter as patients have not met us before, which is unique to this specialty. They are coming into an emergency department, sometimes under the most difficult of circumstances. There is a fear of not knowing. People come in without knowing the extent of the illness or injury they have and may fear the worst. There may be financial factors because this has happened unexpectedly, and there has been no preparation for it, and the extent of the cost may not be known. The patient does not know the physician or staff, and may have been taken to a hospital he or she has never been to before. In that setting an emergency physician needs to be able to establish a relationship of trust and safety. Without safety, people cannot communicate what is really on their minds. A relationship of safety requires a situation in which no judgment is applied to the patient. The physician has to demonstrate an interest in the patient through tone of voice, eye contact, body language, and choice of words. All of these things matter. Other examples are sitting down with the patient and shaking hands or making some type of contact to let the patient know you are there for him. These things in an emergency department are very important.

It's also important to be willing to set aside stereotypes and opinions. Of course, being human, many of us are sometimes unaware that we are harboring or holding various opinions of people. It is very important to set those things aside and listen to the person – and always listen from the standpoint that if something does not make sense initially, you should start from the perspective that maybe the patient is describing something that is new to you or that you're unaware of. So rather than dismissing it, it is much better to think that maybe this is something you are unfamiliar with, and it might be something you need to look into and learn more about. These things can really help you get established with the patient.

Another thing that might seem basic in a way but that is often left out when communicating with patients is illustrated in the following scenario. A patient comes to the emergency department for an injury: He has fallen and broken his wrist. You see there is something else affecting that person's health that might be germane, and you believe it would be important to discuss it with the patient: Your exam shows the underlying problem is alcoholism.

Fifty years ago perhaps the doctor had implicit permission to intrude because the old medical paradigm was one in which the doctor had a highly paternalistic role. The doctor could chide the patient about his drinking problem, admonishing him to stop.

Now, back to your patient who has fallen. Today you cannot have an intrusive conversation with a patient about lifestyle issues or drug or alcohol abuse without obtaining permission. If the patient comes to an emergency department seeking care for a fractured wrist, this person has not necessarily given you permission to discuss alcoholism, and you might be intruding unless you specifically say something that establishes partnership and requests permission to go further. So you might say to the patient, "As your physician I can see something that may be affecting your health that could be part of what is going on here, but I would like to ask your permission to talk to you about it." Most patients will agree to do so. Some patients may say no, in which case I would respect their decision.

People establish boundaries for what they are comfortable with and how far you can explore something, but many patients will allow you to go ahead. I would then say, "I am aware that alcohol is beginning to affect you in ways it has not in the past. I can see from your blood work your red blood cells have become affected." I have actually had situations where patients have stopped smoking as a result of a conversation crafted in this manner in the emergency department. In contrast, if I just went up to a patient and said, "Smoking is bad for your health; you should stop" – as if I were the patient's parent – it's not going to work. On the other hand, if a patient comes in with a deterioration of bronchitis or emphysema, and I say, "There's something I'd like to speak with you about that is affecting your ability to breathe. I am concerned about it and your well-being, and I would like to speak with you as someone on your side" – most people would say yes. If I discuss how I see smoking affecting their oxygen content, and then acknowledge that maybe years ago, when they were younger, it didn't affect them, patients will stop and listen because they see you are on their side, and you have asked permission to intrude.

In an emergency situation when I am meeting someone I have never met before, I need to establish a relationship of trust and safety. I need to ask permission to go beyond what might be considered normal boundaries. I need to demonstrate empathy and concern. And I need to communicate professionalism with every aspect of who I am. That is why it does matter what you look like, because people draw conclusions about you in less than a minute. If I look sloppy, people might conclude my care is sloppy. If my tone of voice sounds harsh, people might conclude I am not caring, even though that may not be true.

We usually do not teach doctors their voices can be used as instruments; yet the power of the human voice is partly why singing as an expression of music is so essential to us. Take Beethoven, for example. An astonishing thing he did, around 1820, was to take the symphonic form, which conformed to a very well established structure at that time, and alter the form to include the human voice. Thus, his Ninth Symphony was groundbreaking and actually revolutionary in its time. But what was behind this startling introduction of the human voice? The need to use the human voice to create a level and complexity of musical expression that Beethoven could not achieve with musical instruments alone. Sound and the human voice are enormously valuable and can be used in healing, but these things are not discussed or taught in traditional science or medicine.

Greatest Challenges

It is increasingly difficult to deliver healthcare in our environment. Tremendous demands are placed upon the healthcare profession and physicians for documentation and compliance with a variety of federal and local accreditation and licensing standards. Maintaining the documentation is very time-consuming. Some of the compliance rules are complex and require fulltime work to understand the laws and create the paperwork and documentation for compliance. This is different from being a doctor. An enormous amount of administrative work is required to deliver healthcare and be a physician. The process of billing is very complicated, and the administrative work necessary to bill takes up a large share of the healthcare budget. A tremendous amount of work and time is required simply to go about the business of accreditation, compliance, and billing.

Being a physician is actually not difficult for most physicians who are trained to do what they do and who do it well. Sometimes people think being an emergency physician must be so stressful for me – to be in an emergency department with serious situations coming in, such as heart attacks and gunshot wounds. Of course not every situation and patient encounter is at the highest levels of acuity and severity; even in the busiest of places these do not happen on a continuous basis. But when patients with life-threatening illness or injury present to the emergency department, I find that for me, I am trained to manage those situations, and when something of that nature comes in, I find myself focused, relatively calm, and clear about what needs to be done. I do not find those sorts of things stressful.

What is very stressful for many physicians is that it is not easy to deliver excellence in healthcare, particularly from a large systems or organizational perspective. In other words, what it takes to actually get your hospital accredited or surveyed successfully, to get your residency training program sufficient educational and teaching resources, to deliver healthcare in urban or lower socioeconomic regions, and to train the next generation of physicians is very difficult in today's environment because there are fewer and fewer dollars available. Furthermore, at the same time, more and more documentation is required to get the shrinking dollars that are out there.

This is a very highly regulated industry, and it is sometimes difficult to be creative in certain ways with management approaches because the regulations may preclude that. So I think it is very stressful for physicians and everyone working in the healthcare professions, including non-clinical personnel such as administrators.

Additionally, I believe physicians want to have the human element as a component of their practice, but cognitive and humanistic skills of physicians are not emphasized in the way in which dollars are allocated for reimbursement. The emphasis by third-party and governmental payers is on compensation for technical procedures. Technology does hold a certain allure and amazement about what can be done. I think it is really miraculous to be able to put a valve into someone's heart, or to provide a hip prosthesis so someone can walk again, or to pass a catheter into someone's blood vessel and open a coronary artery. On the other hand, spending sufficient time with someone to arrive at a difficult diagnosis or opening new perspectives through counseling or therapy can require highly skilled cognitive work and produce equally miraculous changes in people's lives. New approaches to well-being (such as losing weight, stopping smoking, changing to a more active lifestyle, or resolving destructive situations in their personal relationships so their relationships or outlook may be healthier) can have life-long benefits, including reduced use of healthcare resources. That kind of work with patients, which often includes the humanistic elements, however, is not always reimbursed, which means many patients will have decreased access to preventive care, medical counseling, stress reduction, and mental health care.

It is difficult to deliver the excellence in healthcare that everyone is looking for in an environment in which there are decreasing resources and less money. It is easy to say on a national level, "Let's not do so many CT scans," or, "Let's not provide this type of technology," or, "Not everybody needs this level of care." But if it is you personally or your family member, the individual medical care is everything to you. You cannot apply statistics to the individual. If the odds are 100-to-1, chances are it will not happen to you, but if it does, it is everything to you. If you are the one who needs the care, you want what is currently perceived as the best. It is a very difficult thing to ration healthcare to the individual patient standing in front of you.

There is also a great deal of information out there on the Internet, which is certainly going to change healthcare, and already has. People have access to far more information about the outcomes produced by hospitals and physicians. I just finished my survey for the New York state physician database, and people can now look up information about me and my medical background, whether there have ever been actions taken against my license, and so on. With this kind of information out there, people will make more medical selections regarding which hospital or physician they use based on information from the Internet. They will also be able to learn more about diseases. If fewer and fewer dollars will be available, how do you say no to a patient who may have read about a certain test that, at least from their perspective, should be run in their situation?

Numerous other challenges abound, as well. There are major challenges in delivering pre-hospital care by ambulance squads and paramedics. Public funds are decreasing for maintenance of paramedic units, and voluntary squads are not available in all communities. There are major challenges in maintaining the emergency departments around the country. And there are increasing numbers of uninsured or inadequately insured patients. Access to healthcare is limited for many people in our country.

We face significant issues now that are expected to worsen in the years ahead. Most important is that there is a national and even international nursing shortage. Also, the resources and teachers needed to train the next generation of doctors will be a major challenge. There is a national crisis in the medical malpractice insurance industry. Several large national malpractice insurers have either closed or stopped offering malpractice insurance. Significant numbers of physicians in certain specialties, such as neurosurgery, orthopedics, and obstetrics and gynecology, have either stopped practicing medicine altogether or stopped working in certain aspects of their practice, such as obstetrics. It will require a lot of creative work to look at all these areas and develop new solutions.

From a more individual perspective, doctors also face the challenge of staying on top of a rapidly evolving field. I use several approaches to staying current. First, my involvement in a residency program keeps me continuously challenged to stay current and learn new things because my students challenge me to examine things in fresh and new ways. One of the wonderful dynamic tensions is that which exists between the older, experienced physician and the younger resident physician or medical student. The fresh, almost naïve perspective of the younger physicians and students permits them to seek answers and think about possibilities in ways that allow the question, "Why not?" This environment of inquiry and scholarship is reflective of any teaching environment. That keeps me awake to new ideas.

Another approach is to continually read journals, particularly professional journals, because they bring us the latest in scientific developments and analyze things from a peer-reviewed perspective. I also look at textbooks on a regular basis, exchange ideas with colleagues, and am generally willing to rethink things. That is what I mean about not having a hardening of attitudes: to carry a certain quality of innocence or childlike inquiry into one's work and to always be willing to look again and consider not knowing. It's very powerful to consider not knowing. Experience can sometimes be a bad thing, because it can give you the impression that you already know, and then you may not discover something new. I also go to conferences several times a year, and consult with my colleagues around the country.

I seek to keep in touch with my humanity through the impact that art has in the world. It is very valuable to look at art, listen to music, go to movies and theater, and experience all sorts of cultural endeavors. This helps because part of the work of the artist in the world is to have us rethink ourselves and challenge ourselves, and I think art throughout the centuries has forced us to stretch ourselves to think beyond where we currently are. Being in touch with things outside of medicine (such as friendships and culture) helps, as does travel, which exposes us to other countries' ideas about healthcare and well-being. These are wonderful ways to stay fresh and current and to consider new approaches.

Marc Borenstein, M.D., F.A.C.E.P., has been Chairman of the Department of Emergency Medicine of the Newark Beth Israel Medical Center since 1999 and its Residency Program Director since 2000. With 23 years of clinical experience and 19 years of management experience in both urban and suburban teaching and non-teaching emergency departments, he has been actively involved in academic emergency medicine and residency training since 1988.

An associate professor in the Department of Medicine of the Columbia University College of Physicians and Surgeons, Dr. Borenstein also serves as an examiner for the American Board of Emergency Medicine and as a reviewer for Annals of Emergency Medicine and Academic Emergency Medicine. He is the cochair of the Education Committee of the New Jersey Chapter of the American College of Emergency Physicians, as well as cochair of the Sickle Cell Anemia Task Force at the Newark Beth Israel Medical Center.

Dr. Borenstein received his M.D. from New York Medical College, Valhalla, New York, and his B.A. in biological sciences from Columbia College in New York City. He took post-graduate training at the Mayo Clinic, the Norwalk Hospital in Norwalk, Connecticut, and the Stamford Hospital in Stamford, Connecticut.

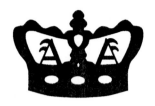

THE COMPASSIONATE PHYSICIAN: STAYING ALIVE IN TODAY'S BUSINESS OF MEDICINE

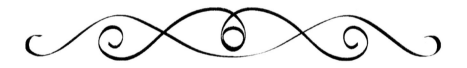

ARTURO CONSTANTINER, M.D.
New York Downtown Hospital

Director of Nephrology and Dialysis

The Importance of Passion and Compassion

Medicine is much more of an art than a science. Although a lot of the data in medicine is based on scientific data and scientific research, every individual is different; therefore it's a science that is far from exact. As a physician you must apply a great deal of common sense and a well-informed interpretation of the scientific data to each individual patient. You have to use clinical judgment and not treat every disease and every patient like a recipe in a cookbook. For example, you really have to know the social condition of the patient. Prescribing medications the patient cannot take or tolerate or afford may represent the use of good scientific data, but it will not be helpful to the patient. Medicine is an art because you have to be creative in how you treat a patient.

The most important quality is to be able to communicate with your patient. It is critical to listen to the patient and talk to the patient at a level that he or she will understand. A doctor should not give a sermon or a speech to the patient; a doctor should try to exchange ideas. A doctor should let the patient talk and not interrupt because many times the doctor will miss some of the symptoms of the patient. The doctor has to be compassionate and available. The doctor must have tremendous respect for the patient, in every sense of the word. A doctor should show care and warmth, and make the patient feel at ease so he or she can be open and disclose necessary information to the doctor. If a physician intimidates a patient, makes him or her feel uncomfortable, or is judgmental, the patient will reserve a lot of information that would be very helpful for the physician's diagnosis.

I admire different types of doctors. I admire a physician who has a tremendous amount of knowledge, but if that knowledge is not combined with human warmth and dedication, then I can't fully admire him or her. My role model is a physician and friend of mine. I don't think I've ever seen her say "no" to a patient or not be available, or not have a kind word or a smile for a patient. She is a physician who is completely devoted to her practice.

The practice of medicine must be pursued with passion. Governmental bodies are currently trying to restrict physicians from working more than 80 hours a week or 24 hours in a row, but the medical profession is far from being a nine-to-five job. While I realize a person under fatigue cannot perform as well as someone who is well rested, one has to understand that in this job you know when it starts, but you don't know when it ends. A doctor cannot lock the door on a patient and say, "OK, I'm on my way out." In a way, medicine has become more difficult, because although technology and drug developments have helped us, we're creating more technicians than people who really know how to practice the art of medicine.

The Doctor-Patient Relationship

A doctor must always be sensitive to the needs of the patient. If a patient has a headache, for example, the doctor should try to gather information about all the symptoms associated with the

165

headache in a brief interview. A headache is one of the most common symptoms that bring patients into the office, and although, fortunately, most headaches have no organic cause, such as a brain tumor or other serious condition, it's important to search for clues that might point to a more serious or systemic disease. You must be sensitive to the anxiety of the patient, because most patients, especially those who have never had headaches and are experiencing a headache for the first time, are probably thinking about the worst-case scenario. We have to be sensitive to their anxiety and preoccupations, while at the same time we have to reassure them that we understand their pain, and that we will go all the way to find the cause of and a treatment for their condition. We have to be sensitive and not alarm the patient unnecessarily. Again, we must make the patient aware that there are certain parts of the physical exam, and maybe ancillary tests as well, that will have to be done to get to the root of the problem.

Today, patients are savvier because of the Internet and the amount of information they have access to. Reading newspapers, books, and magazines, listening to the radio, watching television – all forms of media have made patients more educated. While it is clearly advantageous to have more educated patients, sometimes the information that is spread does not have enough of a basis to make it valid. Sometimes the patient thinks the doctor is doing something wrong or ignoring important information because the patient found some data in the newspaper; this can be frustrating for the physician.

The patient sometimes feels the doctor should be able to respond within minutes of his or her phone call. Although most physicians do try to respond, in many situations it is impossible. In an emergency the doctor will always be available, but the patient should not consider every little situation an emergency. There's a misconception by patients that doctors make them sit and wait unnecessarily in the waiting room. The truth is that the practice of medicine is not something you can plan on a daily basis with a fixed schedule. Emergencies happen, and patients call with needs that must be addressed that day, and the doctor has to schedule those patients on an emergency basis. When a physician makes a patient wait, it is not intentional; it is the result of the unpredictable nature of the practice of medicine.

Some patients also have the misconception that physicians are extremely expensive and exist merely to exploit patients and gain money. Although there may be physicians who practice that type of medicine, most physicians are not in the business of medicine to generate massive profits. Obviously it's an income-producing profession, but if an individual were to choose a profession based on money, he would not choose medicine.

Most people, when calling to make an appointment, have some degree of anxiety; whether they need the attention immediately or not, the patient seeks some relief of that anxiety. My approach is to provide my patients with access to my office almost as soon as they call. I try to communicate with the patient in the best way possible, and to respond to their questions and make myself available by telephone to clarify or expand on the encounter. Many times we think a patient understands everything explained in the office, but often a patient will leave the office and after a few minutes, he or she will become completely confused about what was said or the directions for the medications, primarily due to a high level of anxiety. So a follow-up phone call to clarify instructions, directions, or the diagnosis can be critical.

I try not to bring the patient to the office repeatedly unless it's absolutely necessary. In my practice I personally give my patients their results via telephone; I don't use my secretary for this task. I instruct my patients to reach me within a few days from when their blood test or other tests were ordered. I bring the patient back to the office for a follow-up or a treatment only if we discover a condition detected by the blood tests or other ancillary tests.

Unfortunately, you have to tell some patients – hopefully very few – bad news. In those situations I definitely bring the patient back to the office. A physician should never give bad news over the phone. If I have doubt or fear about results I reschedule the patient to come and discuss them. Occasionally I even make up an excuse – that the blood test was lost and I need to run a new one, for example – just to avoid breaking bad news over the phone. Perhaps because of the culture I come from I find it unethical to break bad news over the phone. In American medicine the usual practice is to be 100 percent open and completely up-front. I find that many times this can be cruel to patients, especially when there's always a possibility that things are not as bad as they initially appear. With many patients a doctor should not tell them they have cancer until they actually have the diagnosis in their hand, with a biopsy. I've found many physicians who, because of the need to be totally up-front, will throw a lot of diagnoses on the table and worry the patient unnecessarily, creating much more anxiety, and then call to say there is good news. I think it's important not to hide information from the patient, but it's also important to avoid alarming the patient; the information should be disclosed in a very smooth way.

I recently made rounds at the Veterans Administration, and to my dismay I found that people were looking at me as a rare animal in the way I approach a physical exam. Unfortunately, younger students and physicians are more used to receiving data and information from lab tests, MRIs, and CAT scans, and the physical exam is in some ways falling by the wayside. One should attempt to catch up with the times and not try to live in the "glory days" of physical exams, but there will never be a substitute for a good history-taking.

Twenty or 30 years ago scientists were trying to develop a computer that would interview the patient. The personal interview reflects the art of medicine. That dialogue between the patient and the physician gives the latter a feel for something that could never be substituted by a machine. We do have to keep up with the times; we can't say, "Things were done this way 40 years ago, so we have to keep doing it," but the patient-physician relationship should not change. I don't like the idea of robot doctors. There is already long-distance surgery, with a surgeon from New York operating on a patient in China, using robotics. The technical part of medicine will change and is changing, but there are certain things that will never change.

The doctor-patient relationship has changed significantly in the past 10 to 15 years, primarily because of managed care. The loyalty of a patient to a physician has changed because every time a patient's insurance changes, he or she has to change physicians. A long relationship of 30 or 40 years between patients and doctors is rare. Doctors also sometimes cannot be loyal to their patients because, for one reason or another, the doctor may decide to stop accepting the type of insurance a patient uses, which will cause a patient to have to change physicians. In that respect the relationship has changed significantly for the worse. This can frustrate the doctor, in the sense that he or she has lost the freedom to refer patients to physicians who are reliable and responsible. Instead, he or she has to use the managed-care "yellow pages" to make a referral. The process is time-consuming for the physician, and he or she will not get the same results or response as from someone the physician knows personally. The patient-doctor-office relationship has become much more difficult, and there is much frustration on all sides.

Managed care has taken away the dollars from the hospitals and the physicians to put them in the pockets of investors and managers. It has not added much to satisfy the patient or the physician. However, the idea of being able to use preventive medicine is fantastic, and managed care seems to implement this practice more than the old type of insurance. Preventive medicine is something we should be looking forward to in the future, especially since we know there are so many ways to prolong life – and I mean by that the quality of life, not the number of years.

The principle of managed care was, in theory, very good, but in practice it's outrageous. Some managed-care companies – especially the capitated ones – encourage you to keep the patient away from your office to make a buck. The selling point is that you get a flat fee per month, whether you see the patient or not. The flat fee does not cover any of the real costs, so you make money by not seeing the patient. When I hear that, my hair just stands up. It was a good way to control inflation in medicine, but medicine, like education, is a field where inflation is difficult to control, especially if you want to be in the forefront of the field. You can't be at the top in medicine and do the most research without spending a lot of money. Something is definitely wrong with the system; 40 million people are uninsured, and I think that's very wrong. .

I am familiar with other countries' approaches to medicine, and I don't find them to be better. Sweden seems to have a perfect system, but that's primarily because of the homogeneity of their society. It wouldn't work like that in the heterogeneous society of the United States. The stories I've heard about England, where people over the age of 60 were not able to have dialysis because 60 was the cut-off age, are astonishing. In some countries you have to wait six months to get a bypass, but you could go to a private physician and get it done within 24 hours.

I think the medical system in America has worked best, but unfortunately it's being eroded and destroyed. Hospitals are experiencing tremendous deficits, especially teaching institutions, and that really curtails the possibility for training scientists in medicine. The only hospitals in America that make money are for-profit private institutions, and those institutions are not interested in research or development; they're interested in the bottom line. The crisis of the deficit of university centers is going to impact the long-term research capabilities of this country.

The Business of Medicine

As in any business, one starts from the premise that the patient comes first. We have to cater to the patient in the best way we can. I emphasize to my staff that they should sometimes put themselves in the patient's position. You have to be sensitive to the anxiety of a patient who waits a long time on the phone with no response, or who sits in the waiting area for a long time, or whose phone call is not returned, or who is not treated with respect. I instruct the people in my office that we're not dealing with a business in which, if you make a mistake on an order or a shipment, it can be corrected. Here we are dealing with disease, with life and death. The margin for error should be zero. That's not to say that we have not made errors, but luckily we've not made any major mistakes. Any physician who has made no errors or oversights is not practicing medicine. A surgeon once told me, "If you've never taken a healthy appendix out of a patient, you've never done surgery." Nowadays, with technology, these errors have been reduced (everyone gets a CAT scan), but to take out a sick appendix, you have to take out a few healthy ones.

172

As in most professions, doctors need to be on top of new developments in the field. I use as many media as possible. Reading a newspaper gives you quick information on what's going on and will update you on new fields and technologies in medicine. An internist has to gather a lot of information. The newspaper is just a summary that provides quick motivation to examine a current trend extensively. Journals such as the *New England Journal of Medicine* or the *Annals of Internal Medicine* have peer-reviewed articles that are very useful.

The Internet also provides a great deal of information about what is going on. Every day there is health news online, describing something new that is being discussed. That doesn't mean you should instantly believe in the new technologies or practices described, but it makes you much more aware of what's going on. There's a program, developed by a nephrologist, that covers most of internal medicine, called Up to Date. Every three months you get a new CD-ROM updating what's going on in the medical field. It's a fantastic program that allows you to see what's happening currently. Textbooks are rather anachronistic because once they are published, the data is three or four years old. The Internet and monthly publications are very helpful in providing volumes of useful information. Attending conferences is also important because the information is being presented as it's being developed.

Many of us, considering the frustration we experience today, might quickly say we would absolutely not recommend that our children go into the practice of medicine. The profession is not as lucrative as it once was; some physicians are barely making enough to cover their overhead. More important, I find the current system humiliating in the sense that physicians occasionally have to contact 800 numbers to seek approval for a medication or a test from people who are completely ignorant of medicine. I once received a call from a managed-care company seeking justification for placing a patient in an intensive care unit. They said the patient had sepsis and was in shock, and the next question was, "Does the patient have an intravenous line?" At that point you know you're talking to someone who doesn't have any idea – you don't get admitted to the intensive care unit with sepsis and shock, and you don't get an intravenous line, so obviously they had a form to fill in to justify the placement.

Even having said that, I think I would still encourage my children to study medicine because the gratification and the intellectual motivation are beyond understanding. You have to be there to understand it. Again, though, I would encourage people to go into medicine only if they really have the passion and the devotion for it. It's not a profession you can do halfway.

If you can satisfy your personal life with your family and interests other than medicine, then you will be able to bring satisfaction and pleasure into the practice of medicine. Every individual makes of their own profession whatever they want; some people who are workaholics feel that working 24 hours of medicine is what gives them pleasure and satisfaction. That's fine, but personally I find that family is very important, and I like to spend a lot of time with my family. I also like to do charity work to complement medicine and give myself personal satisfaction. I think the profession of medicine is the most rewarding of all professions, in terms of the amount of gratitude from patients. A card from a patient, a note saying you've done something well, hearing from a patient that you've saved their life – there couldn't be any more personal gratification.

Medicine is by far one of the most intellectually stimulating careers because you have to keep studying, reading, and attending conferences on a constant basis to keep up with the rapid changes in technology. The intellectual stimulation and motivation are incredible. Not having practiced any other profession, I cannot say that it doesn't exist in other professions, but I think that when you're dealing with human suffering, pain, and anxiety, being able to help someone gives you tremendous personal satisfaction.

The Golden Rules of Being a Doctor

1. Use discretion. As a doctor, you deal with very sensitive information about individuals, and in many respects you have to practice complete discretion and privacy about what you say, where you say it, and how you say it, because you never know who you're talking to and who would find out something.
2. Be respectful to patients. Be sensitive to their needs, feelings, and emotions.
3. Recognize that you are only human. People will always lack information and make mistakes. Do your best, and when you hit a wall, ask for help and advice from other people. Recognizing your shortcomings doesn't minimize you. On

the contrary, it lets you practice better medicine, learn from other people, and, most important, help the patient.

Arturo Constantiner, M.D., F.A.C.P., is the director of Nephrology and Dialysis at New York Downtown Hospital and associate professor of Clinical Medicine at New York University. He is also in private practice in internal medicine and nephrology, with special interest in hypertension and kidney stones.

Dr. Constantiner is a member of the American Society of Nephrology, the International Society of Nephrology, and the New York Society of Nephrology, and is an Honorary New York City Police Surgeon. He is a member of the Board of Governors of Tel Aviv University and a member of the American Friends of the Tel Aviv Sourasky Medical Center.

Born in Mexico City, Dr. Constantiner graduated from the Faculty of Medicine, National University of Mexico. He did post-graduate training in internal medicine at Elmhurst Hospital in New York and a fellowship in nephrology at Mt. Sinai Hospital in New York.

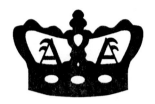

A RELATIONSHIP THAT WORKS: THE DOCTOR-PATIENT PARTNERSHIP

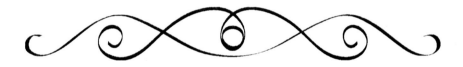

MARTHA S. GRAYSON, M.D.
New York Medical College

Senior Associate Dean for Primary Care

Defining the Art and Science of Medicine

The art of medicine lies in the ability of the physician to individualize patient care. The physician must evaluate the patient's medical condition, his or her beliefs, and his preferences for how things should be done. The physician may have two patients with the same disease, but use totally different methods in treating them. There is also an art to communicating with patients. Some physicians are natural communicators, while others gain this skill with experience. There has been significant research into the art of communication – what works and what doesn't.

The science of medicine involves, first, taking an accurate and objective medical history, followed by a thorough physical examination and, second, knowing how to evaluate information obtained from this assessment and any diagnostic tests. As a doctor, and especially as a primary care physician who takes care of patients with a wide range of medical problems, I cannot reasonably know about every possible diagnostic test or therapy. But, as a scientist, I must know where to find accurate and reliable information, and how to make sound judgments based on the information obtained. Medical schools now acknowledge the importance of this aspect of medicine – it is called "evidence-based medicine." We teach our students early in their medical careers how to obtain and evaluate medical information on prognosis, diagnostic tools, and therapies.

How to Be a Successful Doctor

There are a number of qualities important to being a successful doctor. Certainly, strong interpersonal skills, such as compassion and respect, are critical. A successful physician must be able to look at the many factors that determine how a patient relates to both health and disease, including the patient's culture, background, spiritual beliefs, family relationships, and community. Again, communication skills are critical. The physician needs to explain things clearly. He has to be attuned to the individual's level of understanding about a certain disease or a treatment, and try to communicate at that level.

It's also very important to have strong analytical skills. A doctor cannot think only in terms of black and white; he or she must be comfortable looking at things in different ways and noticing the shades of gray. Another important requirement for success is staying current in one's field. So a certain amount of curiosity and a desire to continue to learn are important. It is imperative that a good doctor follows his or her vision, acts in a professional manner, honors confidentiality, and is kind.

I also believe that a doctor should serve as a role model for healthy lifestyles. I sometimes share tips with patients on how I fit exercise into my daily routine, or remember to take calcium during the day. They appreciate the pointers and like that I practice what I preach. Sometimes as I am walking into the hospital, I see doctors or nurses smoking cigarettes outside the entrance door. This sends a terrible message to our patients. If a health professional is unable to serve as a role model for healthy

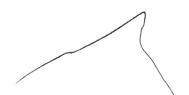

lifestyles, he or she should, at the very least, not publicly flaunt dangerous or unhealthy behavior!

Setting goals and having a timeline are important. It is useful to review your goals and examine what you have accomplished. It may help to make a one-, five-, or even 10-year plan, bearing in mind that none of us can perfectly foresee or control the future. In my profession, working for both a hospital and a medical school, this is a little easier because there are annual reviews that other physicians do of me and I do of others. If I have grants, progress reports, or annual reports to write, I often discuss the goals I have and how I have worked toward them. My personal goals often involve exploring things that are new or different, so I will look at an area that I may want to learn more about. For example, this year I did a leadership fellowship for women in academic medicine, and I learned a great deal about organizational, administrative, and financial skills, areas that are important at this point in my career.

I rely heavily on scheduling; I use the calendar on my personal digital assistant (PDA) for both professional and personal activities. By having my outside interests scheduled in along with my duties as a physician, I keep some time in my life for these activities. Making plans is important to ensure that I have time outside of work, because in medicine, there can always be more to do. I think it's also very important to have a strong coverage system, so I can be comfortable with whoever is treating my patients while I'm away. Additionally, in academic medicine I need coverage for my teaching programs and administrative roles, as well. I need to feel just as comfortable with my coverage for these aspects of my professional life as with the coverage arrangement for my patients. It's really important to take appropriate vacation time. In my position I have a certain number of weeks off each year. After a vacation I come back refreshed, rejuvenated, and once again ready to work.

There is no one way to learn how to be a competent doctor, but there are a lot of new and interesting ways to train our medical students and residents. One innovative approach involves using what is called standardized patients. An actor plays the role of a patient with a certain disease, and the student or resident does the interview. The actor has a checklist of things the student is supposed to do. He gives the student feedback by saying, "You forgot to listen to my heart," or "You put the stethoscope in the wrong place," or "You forgot to ask a key question." It's a role-playing approach to learning how to have a patient encounter, how to take a history, and how to conduct a physical exam.

There are many interesting computerized programs, as well, to complement the standard textbooks. For example, using cases from a computerized program, a student might order a specific test and receive immediate feedback from the program as to whether that test was appropriate. Such a program allows the student to try out and test what he or she learned from a lecture or from reading a textbook.

Further along in training, a student must determine not only the field of medicine he would like to enter, but also the type of career he would like to pursue. There are so many specialties to choose from, from the primary care physician to the super subspecialist. In addition, a doctor can take on so many different roles, including being a clinician, a teacher, a researcher, an administrator, or some combination. Once the new doctor decides on his role, he must determine how to gain the necessary skills to become that type of doctor. For instance, if he wants to have his own practice, he may need to learn how to run an office or develop some business skills. This may call for courses in practice management or a business education. If he wants to pursue academic medicine, he needs to learn more about research or teaching. There are a variety of fellowships and programs to help obtain these skills. In making a career choice it often helps to speak with someone in a similar position, or a mentor.

What separates a "good" doctor from a "great" doctor is that the great doctor sees his profession not as a job or a career, but as a calling. What he or she does in the world is viewed as a mission, or a vision. I think the really great doctors that I know – whether researchers, physicians, teachers, clinicians, or some combination of these – want to make a difference.

I respect doctors who are kind, dedicated, knowledgeable, and organized, and who really see patients for the individuals they are. No two patients are alike, even if they have the same disease. I'm also impressed with the doctors who, in addition to seeing patients (and especially if they're in a full-time practice), contribute to the training of other doctors, medical students, and residents. At my medical school, we have a whole cadre of physicians – hundreds – who volunteer their time training young medical students in their offices. I think it is admirable that, as busy as they are, they volunteer their time to do that. As it turns out, they get something in return. I've studied the effects on the mentoring physicians, and I've found they actually enjoy the practice of medicine more when they have an inquisitive mind in their office asking them questions.

Some practical advice that's been useful to me is to avoid acting as a doctor for family and close friends. A doctor needs a certain amount of objectivity to provide the best care. At the same time, when I see patients I often think, "How would I treat this person if he or she were a family member?"

I advise others not to use medical jargon when speaking with their patients. When working with patients, I also write things down as much as possible. Patients frequently forget many of the things said to them, so even if it's something as simple as the type of over-the-counter pain reliever I prescribe for them, I'll write that information down as a reminder. I like to individualize what I do with my patients and check on their understanding. When we talk about something the patient should do, taking medicine for example, I try to determine if they agree with this approach. Will they really take this medicine? It is important to understand their reaction and how receptive they are to what we are discussing, rather than just telling them to do something.

The Challenges of Being a Doctor

I wish it were possible to create a pill that, when swallowed by the patient, would make them automatically follow a healthy lifestyle. My "miracle drug" would get my patients eating right, exercising, avoiding tobacco, and wearing their seatbelts. With regular use of my "drug," the number and severity of the diseases they might develop would be greatly reduced. That is my fantasy!

But, getting back to reality, one of the major challenges in medicine, particularly for a physician in primary care, is keeping up with the steady stream of new information. Sometimes I feel overwhelmed. But in reality it isn't necessary to know everything. I can always talk with other physicians or gather necessary information as a case arises. If I have questions about the care of a patient, I speak with colleagues, look things up, use the Internet, look in my books – I use many resources. In medicine we have to accept the fact that nothing stands still. Everything changes, and we have to be comfortable with that and devise a strategy to keep up with ongoing change. Teaching, more than anything else, keeps me up to date in my field. The academic side of my career motivates me to stay current and ultimately helps me with patient care. So I am always developing programs or looking up information for my students. I recently took over the directorship of our course on teaching clinical skills, and that has forced me to review all the skills required for performing correct physical exams.

Keeping up-to-date doesn't necessarily mean waiting for a journal to come out – although I do like to see what is being printed in the news, because patients ask about the things they read in the newspapers. I do extensive research for the educational programs I run, and I research issues related to my patients. There are a number of books online that are constantly updated and special programs that analyze and update the literature on selected topics. For example, if a patient is traveling through a country where certain infectious diseases occur, having an online site that is constantly updated is very useful. If there were a sudden outbreak of an infectious disease there, I would know about it right away.

More recently, the economics of healthcare have become a challenge for me. Recent developments have brought us new medical technologies and medications, but all of them come at a price. There are a growing number of uninsured people in the United States, and an increasing number of people who are having a difficult time paying for the medications they need. Another concern is the ever-increasing amount of administrative tasks and paperwork. This adds to the time and cost of caring for a patient.

Any doctor you speak to now will tell you he or she is much more overworked than in the past. The causes are fewer healthcare resources and changes in financing. Physicians who practice full time find it necessary to see more patients, and for briefer appointments. In the academic world physicians who both teach and see patients are spending more time in clinical work to generate the revenues to support their academic work. They also spend more time trying to get grants to support themselves.

One of the challenges in academic medicine is to make certain physicians still have enough time for the training of the next generation of doctors. The knowledge base of our physicians has vastly increased, not just in terms of new technology, but also in the understanding of patients and how to relate to them. We need time to teach all this.

One of the challenges that all doctors face is dealing with a terminally ill patient. How much information should the doctor give to the patient? Is blunt talk in order, or is false reassurance better? I try to take my cue from listening to the patient and talking with the family.

Changes in the Medical Profession

The role of the doctor has changed in a variety of ways. Computers have revolutionized the way we get information. Medical records, laboratory results, and x-rays are available electronically in an increasing number of hospitals and doctors' offices. It is enormously helpful to use the Internet and have computerized texts and journals available to both doctors and patients. In addition, regulations have had a major impact on both the way we practice medicine and the way we train our future doctors.

Another change is that alternative, or complementary, medicine has become more mainstream, and physicians are now more apt to recommend it. Many doctors and patients choose acupuncture or massage therapy, for example, to complement traditional medical therapies.

In addition, more and more patients are taking an increasingly active role in their healthcare. They research their symptoms before coming to the doctor and seek multiple opinions. It is a welcome trend, beneficial to both the patient and the doctor.

I practice in New York City, so I am not sure how much I can generalize, but there also seem to be more patients with fewer family members and less personal support. I see elderly people without anyone to visit them in the hospital or take them home when they are discharged. And many people are isolated, lacking the important family and personal support structures people had in the past. We need to come up with new ways to care for those who do not have the social or family support in their lives to help them when they are ill.

In the next few years I think we'll see a continuation of several recent changes in the field. For instance – going back to computers and the Internet – I am personally trying to improve my skills at using information technology and am constantly seeking advice on how to use new medical programs for both the computer and the PDA. We are now able to carry large amounts of medical information on our PDAs, ranging from dosages, side effects, and interactions of medications, to a listing of our patients' diagnoses, allergies, and appointments. The portability of this information will also lead to new rules and regulations about protection of patient confidentiality.

Within the next few years we should be able to have access to an expert in any area of medicine with the help of the Internet. Some areas of the country are already using telemedicine to allow patients in small towns to be evaluated by a specialist in a large urban center on the other side of the country. For instance, you can hook up a stethoscope to a computer that sends heart sounds to a cardiologist at a distant site, or you can have a local doctor look into the ear of his patient and send that image to a head and neck specialist for evaluation. At this point it is just a matter of learning how to use and become comfortable with these diagnostic tools and technologies.

We will continue to see miraculous strides in patient care with new medications, advanced treatments for diseases, transplants, artificial organs, and so on. We will continue to see state-of-the-art drugs and treatments. I think genetics will also play a bigger role in the future. We will be able to identify patients who are at risk for certain diseases, and improve our counseling and preventive therapies.

On the flip side, all of this new and improved technology challenges us with the question of finance. These advancements inevitably have a cost, and we will have to determine what resources are available for healthcare and how much we are willing to pay. Unfortunately, one can predict that the number of uninsured, the number who lack appropriate access to healthcare and medications, will continue to grow. Our nation will need to address this issue so all individuals can have access to healthcare. Facing the challenge of allocating healthcare resources will be difficult. We will have to make difficult choices about what medical care can be provided and what may need to be curtailed. A large portion of our healthcare dollars are spent during the last six months of a patient's life. We will need to examine what we are doing for our patients who are at the end of their lives, and redirect our energies and resources toward providing pain management and comfort.

Finally, patients will take even more control over their healthcare, because they will have access to so much more information. The old paternalistic role of the doctor will become passé. We will find a much more active, inquisitive type of patient who will want to play a major role in healthcare decisions. The doctor and the patient will become true partners.

The Golden Rules of Being a Doctor

1. The Hippocratic Oath (truly the Golden Rule): Do no harm.
2. Respect your patients.
3. Be honest; practice with integrity.
4. Serve as an advocate for your patients.
5. Have concern and compassion.
6. Be a life-long learner.
7. Be an educator.
8. Make a difference!

Martha S. Grayson, M.D., graduated from Tufts University and earned her medical degree from the Albert Einstein College of Medicine. She completed her training in Internal Medicine through the Social Medicine Residency Program at Montefiore Hospital and Medical Center in the Bronx, New York. In addition, Dr. Grayson completed a Primary Care Faculty

Development Fellowship sponsored by Michigan State University and the Executive Leadership in Academic Medicine Fellowship for Women sponsored by MCP-Hahnemann University School of Medicine.

Dr. Grayson has been in academic medicine throughout her career. She is currently the Senior Associate Dean for Primary Care and Director of the Center for Primary Care Education and Research, as well as associate professor of Clinical Medicine, all at New York Medical College. She has served as both a course director and a teacher for a number of educational programs for both medical students and residents, and has been the principal investigator for numerous educational grants. Dr. Grayson has published research on the effectiveness of these teaching programs in national medical journals, including Academic Medicine and the Journal of General Internal Medicine.

Dr. Grayson is a practicing General Internist and serves as the Chief of the Section of General Internal Medicine at Saint Vincent's Hospital and Medical Center in New York City. She has been selected in listings of top primary care physicians in the Castle Connelly Guide of Top Doctors, New York magazine, and Town and Country magazine. She has been selected a Fellow of the American College of Physicians and has served as the elected president of both the New York City Metropolitan and the Mid-Atlantic Regional Division of the Society of General Internal Medicine.

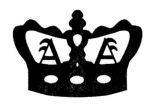

MEDICINE: EMERGENCY ROOM, LOCKER ROOM, BOARDROOM

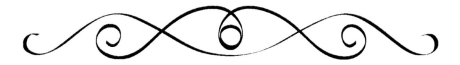

NICHOLAS A. DiNUBILE, M.D.

Hospital of the University of Pennsylvania

Department of Orthopaedic Surgery
Clinical Assistant Professor

Sports Medicine Calling

For as long as I can remember, I always wanted to be a doctor, specifically, a surgeon. My athletic background and my early interest in fitness and exercise pointed me in the direction of the care of athletes. In the late 1970s I saw sports medicine as an amazing new emerging field of medicine. However, when you first start out in practice, you don't necessarily pick and choose what you do; you do a little of everything. I initially did what general orthopedic surgeons do: a lot of trauma and emergency room calls, which involved taking care of broken hips, broken necks, and any number of injuries. Over time, as you develop a reputation and a name, you can focus on what you want to do.

Some people stay generalists for their whole career, but I always had a goal in mind of being very focused on athletes and active people. Part of that drive comes from a very strong parallel interest I have in exercise, fitness, wellness, and prevention. Those interests don't necessarily jive with the crux of what a surgeon is; during my surgical training and in medical school, we were always taught to wait until things break and then fix them. But even before it was in vogue, I was oriented toward prevention, which is fairly unusual for a surgeon. I always had an interest in exercise and taking better care of oneself, and I did a lot of writing and speaking on those subjects early on.

The reason I love sports medicine is that it allows you to combine these interests – you deal with extremely motivated, active people who want to keep going at high levels, even if they get injured or have problems. I found ways to combine all of those interests in one specialty, and I think over time I evolved into also being a knee surgeon, but I also do a lot of educational work nationwide in the area of exercise and wellness.

Early on, when I was in my training as a resident, I started working with the dancers here in Philadelphia – the Pennsylvania Ballet – and when I went into private practice, I became their orthopedic consultant; I've done that for 20 years. Dancers are incredible athletes, and working with them has opened my mind tremendously because they were in tune with a lot of innovative body work that I thought had application to other athletes. They were doing Pilates in the early 1980s, talking about the benefits of massage, and even acupuncture – alternative medicine before it had a name.

When I was a resident, everyone said, "Don't work with dancers. Don't ever take a dancer as a patient – they're crazy. Don't ever operate on a dancer." I can't say how many times I heard that, and I found just the opposite to be true. I found that if you spend the time to let them know you care about their craft and their sport, or their art – whatever you want to call it – and let them know you aren't going to tell them to stop doing it, and that you are going to find ways to keep them going, and if they trust you, they are a tremendous group to work with. Even now, I've found dancers are the most appreciative athletes I work with. They are the smartest; they want to learn more about their bodies; they are interested in prevention; and they have a natural inclination in that direction. From students in dance class to professionals all over the country – even advising Rudolph Nureyev on a foot problem – I've found this to be true.

Zebras and Creativity

There's no question that being a doctor is both an art and a science. In terms of direct patient care, not everything is black and white in science, though we'd like to believe it is. If you read about a certain condition in a medical school textbook, you may assume that's what will present itself every time, but I would say there are more zebras than straightforward black and white situations out there. You have to have a sixth sense; you have to have intuition; and you need to be a bit of a detective. The art is also in communication with patients; if you don't fine-tune that aspect of listening and reading between the lines – between what somebody is saying and what their concerns and fears really are – I don't think you'll be as effective as you can be.

In terms of direct patient care, I think the art is a matter of realizing there will be times when you need to use guesswork and intuition. Hopefully, you will use intelligent guesswork that is driven by your underlying scientific training.

On the other side, creativity is required to innovate. That's not present in direct, one-patient-at-a-time patient care, but it is when you write and try to look at things differently. When I was at Penn, I spent a year researching articular cartilage, which is the surface of joints. We had a chairman who was very excited about research, who said, if you can have one original thought in your life, you're way ahead of the vast majority of people. I think I've had several original thoughts. Many people can be presented with the same information, but you have to see it

NOT MODEST !

differently from everyone else, and that's a creative process. I also like to write; I am working on a new book titled *Body Built To Last,* which will be more for the lay public, and I think it will be very innovative in some of its concepts. It will certainly break new ground. I don't want to write a book that's already been written; I want to do something different. I'm always pushing myself that way.

An example of creativity is that I coined a term a few years ago called "boomeritis," which made national media – just about every TV show and every newspaper, from *The New York Times, The Washington Post,* and the *Los Angeles Times* to CNN, picked up on this, and they continue to use it. I do one or two interviews a week on "boomeritis." Basically, it was just thinking a little more deeply about baby boomers and their aches and their pains, and why that's happening, and how it's a really new phenomenon, and just coming up with a creative, cute name that stuck. The more I thought about it, the more I wanted to write about it, so now I'm writing a book that covers more ground on what happens not only to baby boomers, but to anyone, young or old, who has had their frame fail on them. It's about the "weak links" we all have, or develop, and how to navigate them on the road to staying healthy.

There are always opportunities for creativity. I served on the President's Council on Physical Fitness and Sports under Arnold Schwarzenegger during the first Bush administration. I was a Special Advisor and medical consultant. Way back then – and I don't think this was my unique idea, but the way I developed it was unique – I helped develop and pioneer the concept of "exercise as medicine." That is, doctors need to look at exercise the way they would any pharmaceutical product, because of its powerful effects on the body. We recommended teaching it in medical school, and I can remember writing very creatively, many times, on that topic, just trying to get people to think a little bit differently about something so obvious.

The science side is every bit as important. With evidence-based medicine, you have to be vigilant about looking at studies and determining what is correct and what isn't. You can't just go on intuition or say, "This is how we've always done it, so this is how we'll keep doing it." You have to listen to science, but realize science isn't always right. You need well-designed studies, and you need them to be repeated, flawlessly and without bias. You have to always understand that scientific process. It helped that I spent time in a research lab, where I learned to critically analyze research and studies – to determine what is and what is not a good study, to know what needs to be repeated, and to know how you make a study better – and then learn to apply that information to direct patient care.

Science actually should drive everything you do. Even though I am open-minded – more so than the average orthopedic surgeon in terms of alternative medicine, chiropractic care, and other nontraditional interventions – that does not mean that at some point those alternative techniques should not be proved scientifically. If you take care of patients and make recommendations, at some point you have to look critically at what's being done and be willing to talk to patients about it. Every week, it seems, some new study is coming out that denies what was said the week before, but when the evidence starts becoming very clear, and the science gets strong, you really need to adjust what you're doing – but always stay tuned. George Bernard Shaw once said, "Science becomes dangerous when it imagines that it has reached its goal." Medicine should always strive to be a more perfect science.

Defining Success as a Doctor

Success depends on the specialty you choose; in some specialties in medicine, you never come face-to-face with a patient. For a pathologist, for example, many of your patients are no longer living, and there is little if any direct patient care, so I don't know that you need great interpersonal communication skills in that setting. But for doctors who work with patients – and that's the majority of us – success comes only with a caring attitude.

You have to care; you have to be willing to work very hard and put your profession and your patients first. Fame and success, especially as a surgeon, come to a doctor who knows how to communicate. The word "doctor" comes from a Latin word that means, "teacher," and I think a doctor is a teacher first. I come from a family of teachers, and I think that's where I may have picked up some of those skills. It's not something you learn in medical school; you either have it, or you don't. You can always improve it, but some people are just more natural. You need that combination of communication skills and, obviously, the technical side. You can't just talk a good game; you also have to be, as a surgeon, very good technically. My area of expertise, arthroscopic knee surgery, requires an almost video-game mentality and agility with good 3-D skills. But if you can put those two things, the interpersonal and the technical, together I think you'll be one of those standout doctors, or what they call the best.

Because my practice is so specific in terms of the surgery I do (*i.e.,* knee surgery and arthroscopic surgery), half the patients who call my office wind up having me refer them to someone else. People trust me; I get calls from people from around the country asking me for advice on whom they should see for certain orthopedic or even medical conditions.

Whenever I recommend a doctor – whether it's an orthopedic surgeon, an internist, or any other kind of surgeon – for me to give a strong recommendation I need to see two qualities in a doctor. They have to be knowledgeable and technically very good as a surgeon – that's a given, but it's only one side of the coin. Before I recommend them highly I also want to know they will treat that person nicely in the office. That goes beyond just face-to-face communication – they need to be considerate, caring, and professional. I want a doctor who's not going to have people sitting around for two or three hours and not spend time with them, not look them in the eye, not answer all their questions, and be too rushed. That's a challenge for all of us in today's managed care–driven healthcare environment, but I still think it can be done. I look for knowledge and technical skills, but I also want them to treat people nicely, as they would a member of their own family or a loved one.

Sometimes I'll tell a patient, "Look, I know this individual is a great surgeon, but I don't know how well he's going to treat you," so I don't give him the big two thumbs-up; I just give him one thumb-up. There are times when that might not matter; if you have a brain tumor and you want the best brain surgeon, for example, I would say, "Don't look for this guy to be your best friend, but take his technical expertise." In some instances you don't need that best friend, but I think any time you are ill, a little hand-holding and compassion can go a long way. I believe it influences the healing process, patient satisfaction, and ultimately your outcomes.

I believe you can influence your patient's attitude, and I believe their attitude affects their healing and recovery. The more you talk to them up front, and the more their expectations are set properly about what will happen and what degree of success they can expect to have after a surgery or other intervention, the more likely they will be a happier patient afterward. I think outcomes are fueled by patient expectations, and I think that's one place where doctors don't do the best job. Some doctors don't spend the time to let people know what to expect, so no matter how well the patient seems, even if the doctor says they're doing great, if they are not doing as well as they thought they would, they will not be happy.

The best advice for doctors is to put the patient first. I try to treat a patient as I would if he or she were one of my relatives – my mother, my sister, a best friend. Quite often you see surgeons who do a certain kind of surgery, but when their own relatives get sick, they don't necessarily recommend it right away; they have a double standard. I try to treat everybody well, and I try not to necessarily act in terms of what's best for me economically. With many patients it's like a friendship that you develop over the years, where they really trust you. I make my living doing surgery, so when I talk patients out of surgery, they are somewhat surprised, but there's a level of trust that comes right away.

In terms of being a successful surgeon, one of my teachers gave me a different kind of advice that I have found to be very true but not often taught: "When you're in your training, you learn how to operate. Afterward, with a little bit of experience, you learn when to operate, which is the indication of whether you're using the right surgery at the right time." It's not just a matter of whether you can technically do it; it's really about making the decision when it is appropriate.

"With experience, you learn the most important thing, which is when not to operate." That takes a bit of a learning curve, because when you're finished with medical school and your residency, you're very enthusiastic, and you think you can cure everybody with your talent and your knife. At that point you have to realize there are some things you're probably better off not meddling with, that you actually can make people worse, and that complications can affect the suitability of surgery. Unless you're clear that the odds are very heavily in favor of tremendously helping someone, then maybe you're better off passing on it, even if they're looking for surgery. Many patients come in looking for more surgery, and it's not easy to sit down with them and say no, because you know some of these patients will go to one of your colleagues and get the surgery anyway. It takes restraint, but if you put the patient first, the decision-making gets easier

Balancing Personal and Professional Lives

Unfortunately, I may not have done the best job in balancing my personal and professional lives. I grew up in a house on Broad Street, the busiest street in downtown Philadelphia, and my uncle was an orthopedic surgeon named Frank Mattei. We had a three-story brownstone, and his office was on our first floor, so there was a doctor in my home where I grew up, and I interacted with him, and he influenced me tremendously. Maybe directly or indirectly, I learned some things there. I saw a guy who worked day and night, who worked endlessly, who put his career before anything else. To me it was very exciting back then, that he'd have to go out in the middle of the night all the time and take care of people who were badly injured. He helped so many people. These days I would cringe if I had to do that every night! But at that time in my life, it motivated me.

Your reasons for becoming a doctor change as you stay with it; I have different reasons now for loving it. Interestingly, the things that drew me to the profession originally are not the things that make me love it now. I think I realized through my uncle what kind of commitment a career in medicine took. I knew from the start that I would have to wait until I was really set in medicine and when I was really the best I could be, before I could put anything like marriage first. Unlike a lot of my friends who got married early and had a lot of struggles balancing a family and a marriage with a more-than-full-time profession like medicine, I waited until I was in my forties to get married. I just turned 50, and I am blessed with wonderful children whom I can put first, because I'm established and I'm not running out every night for a meeting or in the middle of the night with emergency calls; I really can devote my time to them. *When did you have time to screen your wife?*

But short of them, I really think my own personal life outside of my family does suffer. I have very little leisure time outside of my family, and the little leisure time I have I put to working out, exercising, and staying healthy. I spend hardly any time with my friends, and that is something I really need to work on. In the past I skied and played tennis, but I've found there's only so much room, and if you want to be the best in your field and a great family person, that creates a challenge for your other personal needs. *only the best. Mr. Macho.* *Then let me tell you something you don't have. any friends.*

oh brother

During the 76ers basketball season, things really get tight in terms of time. Caring for pro athletes is a major commitment. So I try to find ways to do the things I like with my family, and that becomes my fun stuff. Again, you try to figure out ways to do it, but in my instance, focusing 100 percent on my career early on, before marriage, was a wise choice. My family can now be my number one priority. What gets me into trouble is that I don't just see patients, teach, and have my family; I have many outside interests, and I do a lot of media-related work – TV, print, and Web. I would say I'm one of the few most quoted doctors in America, if not the most quoted doctor in America. I do three or four major media interviews a week. A lot of that is because I am

Good grief. He's also one of the biggest prima donnas!

interested in educating the public, and I've developed a good name for that with the press. That takes a different set of communication skills and a real understanding and sensitivity to the reporters' needs and deadlines. I get calls all the time from national sources, and I find it very rewarding to help influence so many people. The power of the media for health is really untapped, and I think we are entering a new era with the Internet. I also like to write, so it gets tough – there's certainly not enough time and way too many time vampires. I wish the days were longer, or I didn't need to sleep.

you ever been ill?

Just Damn!

what an A-hale.

How old is this guy?

50. oh yeah.

He has midlife crisis.

Staying on Top of the Game

Staying on top of medicine is a never-ending process. I trained in a very academic, high-intensity program at the University of Pennsylvania. The orthopedic program there is one of the highest-ranked programs in the world, and I can tell you that within a few years of finishing there, we were no longer practicing the same things I learned in my residency. There are always new things, and you have to be vigilant about what you need to read and about learning new techniques, technology, and information, especially in your own specialty.

I also try to keep a broader perspective, not only across my specialty but also in other areas of medicine and general health; I try to keep up with what's going on. Of course, it's impossible to be a true expert on everything. That's why I think being a specialist or a subspecialist is positive in that I can know everything in my field. There's virtually nothing I'm not current

oh surely not.

on regarding the knee, and I can embrace even new technology as it is emerging, and I can understand it and build on what I've already learned. It is a building process; technology evolves and gets better, but you don't have to necessarily throw out your old knowledge; you change it slightly, modify it, and add to it. Staying current, if you do it regularly, is not a painful process. It's really an exciting process.

In many instances I feel I've contributed to medicine from a creative standpoint. I enjoy innovating and looking to the future. I consider myself a very creative person; I came into medicine always wondering if I would miss the other things I loved in life, which were music, writing, and the arts. But I think I've found some ways to include the creativity in what I do as a physician. I don't think all physicians can say that, but I think I've found ways to blend that.

Orthopedic surgery is one of the most exciting fields to be in right now because of the technology explosion. Tremendous things are happening now or are around the corner. The future is very bright in our field, and it's very exciting. That's one of the things that motivate you to keep going when the day-to-day work can get pretty tough and sometimes frustrating. In my field, especially in knee surgery, I think one of the things that we're just making breakthroughs in is that when your joints are damaged, there's never been a way to repair them. Even Hippocrates said that when our articular cartilage – the surface of your joints – is damaged, it will never repair; it will only deteriorate. That was true until recently. We now have some new technology that allows us to actually grow cells and resurface certain areas of joints that are damaged.

One thing that will evolve is repairing larger areas of damage, which will allow us to treat – and possibly for the first time halt or reverse – arthritis. In arthritis you have more general damage throughout the area, not just in a focal area. The new technology, whether it's cell technology, such as growing your own chondrocytes and transplanting them, or some of the genetic therapy that's out there, will dramatically alter the future approach to musculoskeletal disorders and even the aging process. New technologies in dealing with both joint surface damage and tendon damage are unbelievably exciting areas in orthopedics. There are new lubricants we're putting into joints – an area called viscosupplementation, for example. Synvisc is a product you can use instead of injecting cortisone into the joints. It's a lubricant you can actually put into the joints and have arthritic joints function more normally.

Researchers have actually come up with a disc prosthesis – an artificial disc for back problems. Joint replacements are becoming more and more sophisticated. We are doing major knee ligament reconstructions thru the arthroscope with minimal down-time and rapid recovery. Our field is exploding with innovative technology.

When you look at the aging population, musculoskeletal care is a major portion of their issues. Right now we spend a trillion dollars on healthcare, and musculoskeletal care is 15 percent of the healthcare dollar – that's staggering. As our population ages that's only going to increase. There will be more people with arthritis, osteoporosis, tendon problems, and bad backs, so it will be great to have more options for them. But it's so much better if you can prevent these things from happening.

With osteoporosis, it's great that we have new drugs to build bones in 70 year olds, but it really starts when you're a teenager, drinking milk and exercising. If you can go into your older years with good bone stock, you won't have problems. We have a generation of kids coming up now that worry me because they're not taking care of themselves. They're not taking calcium, and they're not exercising. At the national level we really need to focus on ways to move people in the right direction in terms of caring for themselves and employing preventive measures. We haven't been able to introduce these things in a widespread enough manner that their effectiveness might allow us to need less high-tech interventions down the line.

The Future of the Medical Profession

Yogi Berra once said, "The future isn't what it used to be," and that is certainly true in healthcare. The "power base" that physicians once had, and perhaps took for granted, has slipped tremendously, and I believe medicine and the healthcare of our nation will pay the price for that. I never thought doctors should be deified, but I also believed that we are and must always be a critical part of the bigger-picture decision-making process, and that is no longer the case. It's unfortunate because there is no greater patient advocate in the whole process than the physician.

I personally know of no harder working, more honest group than physicians, but we as a whole have let things slip dramatically on the administrative and business sides. The insurance companies have taken much more control; the government has stepped in; the hospitals have consolidated and formed large systems; and they have all developed much more power, to the detriment of the individual physician. Just looking back to Hillary Clinton and her ambitious healthcare reform efforts, I do not believe there was a single practicing physician on that panel, or at all involved in that process. That says it all, in many ways. I do believe healthcare is a team effort, but physicians need to re-assume their role as captain of the team, not a bench player.

On the other hand, the whole system would come to a stop without doctors, so we as physicians and our organizations that represent us need to realize we do have tremendous power and tremendous clout. We can't be replaced by a robot or a computer or the latest clinical guideline or pathway, where anybody can figure out what to do for a given patient or ailment. At the same time, we have to be smarter about how we use our power, and we probably can then regain some of the ground we have lost. Doctors must be willing to stand up for themselves and really fight for what is right and what is fair. Unfortunately, that does not happen too often. This power shift has also affected the reimbursement side, because, as private practitioners in this country, we're still the most easily squeezed from an economic standpoint, and I think that will happen further as we go into the future. The little bit of control we got on healthcare spending in the 1990s has now stopped, and we're looking at double-digit inflation in healthcare spending, which could be 17 to 18 percent of our GDP by 2010. I don't think our government will allow that to happen, and when they try to squeeze costs, doctors are the easiest targets because insurance companies, hospitals, and pharmaceutical companies are so powerful. That's why we've seen in the past five years that all of the increases in healthcare spending have gone into insurance company profits, hospital systems, or pharmaceutical companies; whereas physician reimbursement has dropped a little more each year, while overhead expenses continue to rise dramatically.

For example, because of the out-of-control legal system and escalating jury awards, medical malpractice rates have soared to such unaffordable levels that doctors are moving from certain states or going out of business. I believe that if we do not immediately tackle this problem on a national level, the high-quality healthcare we have all come to take for granted will be in jeopardy. There are so many pressures – I wish we could just focus on caring for patients – it really would be better for everyone involved. But those days are over.

In any industry, power shifts occur with time. In professional sports at one point the owners have control, then all of a sudden the athletes have the power. In movies and entertainment the big studios were very powerful at one point, and then the power shifted to the talent – the actors, actresses, and unions. Every industry goes through this, and things will change – it's just a matter of riding things out. I believe many physicians felt we were immune to these types of changes. Things should improve over time, but I think things will get worse for physicians before they get better.

I think we will see more of a challenge, where more and more people are trying to get profit from and take control of what we as physicians do and take a little more power from the physicians. Even though physicians earn maybe only 15 to 17 percent of the healthcare dollar, we actually control 80 percent of it with our pens and with our recommendations, so through what we order, how we write prescriptions, what tests we send people for, and when we put patients in the hospital, we really still control the healthcare spending, and we need to be more accountable for it. That is an area where physicians need to step up and assume more responsibility, both fiscally and from a leadership perspective. That would be an important first step in regaining control of an out-of-control situation. Government pressure would decrease, and the role of managed care would be questioned and decrease. I don't think it will happen in the next five years, but I hope that in the next 10 years we will find ways to be more efficient with the limited resources we have.

In private practice right now, in my office, not a day goes by when my decision-making ability is not questioned or stepped on receptively by someone – usually someone without training in my specialty. I will want to prescribe a drug or other remedy, and they don't cover it, or I need pre-authorization – it really is very frustrating. I am not saying that some degree of it is not warranted, because we as a profession, as doctors, have not been able to be accountable and police ourselves – it's not something we were ever taught to do or expected to do in our training. We were just trained to take care of patients and be knowledgeable about patients; we never really knew the economic side or the business side of it. That is changing, but for now someone else is stepping in to do it, though I believe it is not always in the best interest of the patient. I hope we can step up and be more accountable and look at our own colleagues and say, "You're doing too much of this; the success rates aren't there." We need to look at outcomes, be able to really measure quality, and reward quality.

I hope that a decade from now we will know who the better doctors are and be able to reward them. I also hope we will find the problem ones who are running up the costs by not doing what's right, or making the wrong decisions, and try to educate them and make them better. If they can't get better, then maybe they shouldn't be doing it. I take a rather hard stand on the issue, but I would love to see quality rewarded, and no one really does that now.

It's easy to talk about quality – but much harder to accurately measure it. For a decade I worked part time with the largest healthcare insurer in the world, and I spent a lot of time thinking about how you measure quality in my own specialty. It's not that sophisticated yet; it's still primitive, but I have many ideas, using emerging technology to really measure and improve quality, as well as reduce medical error. With information systems, physicians are getting better at collecting their data and becoming more critical of their data. This is one of the positive results of the revolution we're going through right now; maybe we'll be more accountable, and maybe we'll be better at using information systems and monitoring what we're doing, and really looking at those best practices and rewarding them.

The way things are going, we are spending almost a trillion dollars on healthcare annually, and with inflation we can't keep doing that. There is tremendous waste in the system, and I'll be the first to admit that there is some unnecessary surgery, unnecessary care, and unnecessary duplication of services just because we're not all on the same page. I believe this is changing now in a positive direction. I am convinced that computers, handhelds, and the Internet will play a huge role in the next decade. They will become an integral part of the patient encounter, like the stethoscope or prescription pad. Physicians do embrace technology, but have not yet found effective ways to bring it to the patient's bedside or into the office setting to improve patient care. Our workflow is so different from those of other businesses that it has been a major challenge to incorporate this technology. I hope to do some very creative things with my Web site, drnick.com, which is dedicated to "keeping you healthy in body, mind, and spirit" – again, finding creative ways to improve people's health.

HA

Magic Bullet Fantasies

One thing I would do, if I could snap my fingers and create whatever wonderful drug I would like, is create an immunization to give to children that would prevent them from having any disease or problem until they are well into adulthood. I have a big soft spot for a child with an illness; it just touches me. I think it's unfair. I question everything when I see kids suffering from unbelievable things like cancers or heart disease at young ages. It's unfair for them and impossible for their parents. Instead of a

211

drug that would cure diseases, I would create that immunization so that children could enjoy their youth without having to deal with those awful issues.

For the second drug I would create, instead of a specific drug for one particular ailment like cancer or heart disease, I would create one that would slow down the aging process, because if we can do that, science will do the rest. I firmly believe we're on the verge of a lot of great things in terms of maintaining and repairing the human frame, so if we just keep people from falling apart at a certain age, we could do a lot. People may be living longer, but they are not necessarily living stronger. Unfortunately, we become confined, less active, and less independent. No one wants to live long if they're not going to do well. Dr. Ernst Wynder once said that it should be the function of medicine to have people die young as late as possible. It's not enough just to make people live more years if those years are not quality years. It's also been said that we live too short and die too long. If there were a pill that would slow down or halt the aging process, science would catch up and find the other pills or interventions for cancer, heart disease, and other diseases. Also, in my own field, I would create a new drug that would reverse arthritis and joint wear.

The Challenges of Being a Doctor

Many challenges face physicians today. From a management or business standpoint, the current environment we're working in is a major challenge with managed care, the government, and just about everybody else trying to tell you, the physician, what to do. It's funny that the insurance companies want to be doctors, and they want the doctors to assume the financial risks for the care of the patients. That was managed care's founding tenet – you get paid a certain amount; you take care of a population; and if you spend more caring for those individuals, you lose the money. I think it's very odd that they want us to be the actuaries and the insurance companies, and they want to tell us what to do from a medical standpoint.

I don't think this arrangement is in the best interest of the patient. I'd like to see it go back the other way, where doctors are accountable, but they make the medical calls, and the insurance companies use every ounce of business knowledge and all of their information technology to write fiscally sound policies and help monitor the quality and outcomes of the care rendered with the goal of constantly improving the care delivered.

If you leave an academic position or a salaried, large-group, managed-care type of environment to start a private practice, you need to be both smart and patient. You can't build a private practice overnight; you really have to put time into it. It is especially tricky these days, where you see that the big insurers have consolidated, and so have the hospitals and even many medical practices. I don't think it's a guarantee that doctors by themselves are going to do well – it's just a scarier field out there alone. I'm not sure I would wholeheartedly recommend it now, unless you're very unhappy in your group setting, and you have a loyal group of patients and some funding for your private practice. Most doctors coming out of medical school are in tremendous debt. The residents I work with are $150,000 to $200,000 in debt, some of them even more. Depending on what city you go to, particularly as a specialist, you may face extremely high malpractice rates your first year. It's pretty scary because you'll probably have to take out even more loans and possibly put up some collateral, and it's not guaranteed that you'll make it. Now that's not true of every area in the country, but these are things doctors never had to think about before.

You used to be able to go wherever you'd like – in the city, in the country, in an academic setting – and if you were good and willing to work hard, you would do well. That's not a given anymore. I've seen it in my area, Philadelphia – one of the national hotbeds for malpractice suits – even very top-notch doctors are leaving. The economics are squeezing them; they can't get malpractice insurance, or they can't make their overhead, and I'm talking about the best of the best. I don't think we've ever seen this problem in medicine before. It's a reality that doctors will have to face until things improve.

Another challenge for patient care that I find personally in my specialty is that you can't fix or cure everything. Most of us really want to do that, and I think the general public each year has higher and higher expectations of what medicine can do for them. They want to put the ball in our court and have us solve all their health-related problems. I always find that to be a volley back and forth, where I try to pass the ball back to the patient. People can do so much for themselves, and one big challenge is how to get people to take responsibility for their own health and healthcare, to take better care of themselves, and to get more interested in prevention. All too often patients are in the mindset of "If it breaks, fix it," or "If I get sick, you make me better." We could do much better – from insurance companies to the medical profession, to the government – at putting the onus back on the individual. There are many good reasons for that; the trillion dollars we're spending for healthcare is rising dramatically – double-digit inflation for healthcare spending – yet only about 1 percent of those dollars actually goes to prevention.

At the turn of the last century, back in 1900, we were living only to age 46, and the three leading causes of death were basically out of our control – almost like getting hit by lightning. Pneumonia was the number-one cause; tuberculosis and gastrointestinal disorders were up there, too. These things just came out of the blue, and if you were unlucky, you died. Now we're living to almost 80, and the three leading causes of death have direct links to lifestyle: heart disease, cancer, and stroke. Some experts say that significant percentages – 50 percent to 60 percent of death and premature death in our country – are lifestyle-related. Yet we have not shifted to a prevention strategy.

We will never cure healthcare spending if we keep paying for a disease after it happens, because treating the disease will only get more expensive. The new procedures, the new technology, the new drugs – none of them are cheaper than the old ones, as you can probably see with pharmaceutical companies or instrument companies or devices we put into people getting more and more expensive. With baby boomers aging – getting back to "boomeritis" – we have a huge demographic who are starting to hit their 60s, and when they start getting into more serious health problems, I think we'll see an unprecedented strain on healthcare resources. If you think the elderly consume a lot of resources now, wait until these baby boomers start getting sick, because even with their minor ailments, they are showing an unprecedented ability to consume healthcare resources. When they really get sick – I'm not talking about a sore knee, but heart disease, cancer, and serious diseases – there will be a tremendous strain on the system.

One of these days we have to turn around and say, "It's lifestyles that are driving this, so how do we give people incentives to take better care of themselves?" How do you reward those who do, and how do you at least question those people who seem to not care at all and then want someone else to pay for it – whether by drinking and driving, not wearing a seatbelt, smoking, or unhealthy diets? At some point patients and people need to become more responsible. That's how we'll have a healthier population.

It's unusual for an orthopedic surgeon to be writing about this, given that they usually say, "Call me when the bone's broken," but I really have spent my whole life trying to work out this problem. Somehow my mind got opened to all this. I think one of the things that helped me out was that I had a background in martial arts and an interest in Eastern philosophy. In old China they paid the physician as long as the patient was well, and when the patient got sick, they'd stop paying. There was a huge focus on prevention.

when did you have the time? [handwritten margin note]

With the Eisenhower Foundation I was a special ambassador to China on a sports medicine exchange during the early 1980s. I got to spend a month there to see firsthand the use of many alternative techniques that hadn't hit here yet – whether it was barefoot doctors, acupuncturists, or moxibustion. It's a wholly different approach to healing, and having the martial arts background going into that – I spent a lot of time not just doing martial arts but learning about their philosophy and reading Eastern thought – probably helped open my mind a bit. Also my physician-executive background and experience with a large health insurer allowed me to think more about populations rather than individuals in terms of healthcare. It's a much broader view of what's great about our healthcare system, and also its shortfalls. Making a decision that potentially affects millions of people, instead of just one, is a mind-opening and mind-altering experience.

My work as a Special Advisor to The President's Council on Physical Fitness and Sports during the first Bush administration also broadened my perspective. Our chairman, Arnold Schwarzenegger, was a tremendous leader with a track record for getting things done. Our charge was to improve the health of all Americans. I gained tremendous perspective on what it takes to substantially change health habits and health behaviors across a wide and varied population. All of these types of experiences shifted my perspective and influenced me dramatically.

The Golden Rules of Being a Doctor

Primum Non Nocere: First, do no harm. I think that's a golden rule that fits into everything you do. You put the patient first. Though it's hard because you're pressed for time, you have to remember that each patient is first a person, and they are often intimidated when they are interacting with you, the physician. They may not hear or remember everything you tell them – you must check with them frequently.

Making the diagnosis and knowing what to do or what to recommend is the easy part, often accomplished in minutes or less. The real challenge, and where time must be spent, is pealing away the layers to expose their true concerns and questions and determining what treatment best fits their mindset and situation, rather than your preferences. Also, your expectations and definition of success with treatment or interventions may differ widely from your patient's. It's about reaching people and ultimately trying to have a positive impact on their lives.

The best litmus test is to imagine a loved one in the patient's place, with another physician. What quality and quantity of interaction would satisfy you? To me, the technical expertise and knowledge are givens; you have to have that to be the best. But other qualities, such as caring and communication, become very important in terms of being a truly effective doctor.

A commitment to excellence and caring drives me, and if I try to instill anything into doctors, it's that they need to have that commitment, not just to the patients, but also to nurses and the people around them. You are only as good as the teams you build and nourish. You can't do it all alone; you have to find ways to work effectively with the people around you.

The true leaders I have encountered, in all walks of life, accomplish great things by bringing out the best in others, pointing them in the right direction, and keeping them loyal and motivated. In healthcare this can be a major challenge. In the OR it's rather easy if they give you the same team every time, or the same group of people to work with, and if they sincerely like you, they will perform for you. But it gets harder and harder at a big hospital or university. You have to depend on everyone, from the laboratory to the floor nurses to the administration. When it gets to that point, it's difficult to predictably control all that. That's where true leaders emerge to make a difference. It's easier to arrive at a destination when you are all on the same map with common goals. If your compass is set to "putting the patient first" and "doing no harm," you will never go off course.

Dr. Nicholas DiNubile is an orthopedic surgeon specializing in sports medicine in private practice in Havertown, Pennsylvania. He is also Clinical Assistant Professor of the Department of Orthopaedic Surgery at the Hospital of the University of Pennsylvania. Dr. DiNubile served as special advisor and medical consultant to The President's Council on Physical Fitness and Sports during the first Bush administration, with Arnold Schwarzenegger as Chairman. Additionally, Dr. DiNubile serves as Orthopaedic Consultant to the Philadelphia 76ers basketball team and the Pennsylvania Ballet.

Dr. DiNubile graduated from Saint Joseph's University, where he was president of the student body, and received his medical degree from Temple University School of Medicine. He completed his internship in surgery and his orthopedic residency at The Hospital of the University of Pennsylvania, where he also did basic science and clinical research in the preservation and storage of articular cartilage.

Dr. DiNubile is a spokesperson for the American Academy of Orthopaedic Surgeons (AAOS) and the American Orthopaedic Society for Sports Medicine (AOSSM). He has been chosen one of the "Best Doctors in America" and featured on Good Morning America, CNN, and National Public Radio, and in The New York Times, The Wall Street Journal, The Washington Post, Newsweek, and numerous other publications.

Dr. DiNubile's work has been recognized by several organizations, including the AAOS and AOSSM, for which he is the national representative to the U.S. Department of Health and Human Services' "Healthy People 2000 & 2010" projects. In 1993 he was the recipient of the prestigious Healthy American Fitness Leaders (HAFL) award, given to individuals who have, through their work, improved the health of our nation. Dr. DiNubile has also been a member of the editorial advisory board for The Physician and Sportsmedicine, Muscle & Fitness, Shape, Men's Fitness, and The American Journal of Medicine & Sports.

As Associate Medical Director and Chairman of Aetna U.S. Healthcare's Orthopaedic Surgery Specialty Advisory Committee, Dr. DiNubile helped set national policy for one of the largest healthcare companies in the world. He is a member of the American Academy of Orthopaedic Surgeons, American Orthopaedic Society for Sports Medicine, Arthroscopy Association of North America, American College of Sports Medicine, American College of Physician Executives, and National American Fitness Leaders.

Dr. DiNubile serves as National Medical Advisor for Arnold Schwarzenegger's Inner-City Games, and Chairman of the Inner-City Games in Philadelphia. From 1993 through 1995 he also served as the medical consultant and editorial advisor to "Ask Arnold," Arnold Schwarzenegger's syndicated column in USA Weekend magazine.

Dr. DiNubile is the author of The Exercise Prescription and was on the review panel for The Surgeon General's Report on Physical Activity and Health. He was also editor of Exercise is Medicine, a series in The Physician and Sportsmedicine. Dr. DiNubile lectures and consults nationally on topics of sports medicine, health, and fitness, as well as a variety of healthcare issues.

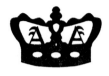

Subscribe to Aspatore

Your One Stop Business Intelligence Source, Based on Your Customized Business Intelligence Profile

Aspatore is the largest and most exclusive publisher in the world of C-Level executives (CEO, CFO, CTO, CMO, COO, Partner) from the world's most respected companies. Aspatore empowers professionals of all levels and industries with first hand, C-Level intelligence and provides this information in the form of books, briefs, reports, essays, articles, and desk references. Information comes straight from top industry insiders, not third party authors and columnists, so the information is pertinent and direct. Aspatore uses Business Intelligence Profiles™ (questionnaires to learn more about each reader) to provide our readers with custom business intelligence that specifically fits their individual needs. Aspatore is your filter to learn more in less time. Be a thought leader, keep your edge, and close more sales. Subscribe to Aspatore.

For Individuals

A) <u>Your Own Custom Book Every Quarter</u>

Receive 4 quarterly books, each with content from all new books, essays and other Aspatore publications that fit your specialty area. The content is from over 100 publications (books, essays, journals, briefs) published every quarter on various industries, positions, and topics, and available to you months before the general public. Each custom book ranges between 180-280 pages and is based on your Business Intelligence Profile (the one page questionnaire you fill out describing the type of information you are seeking that is in the business reply envelope). You can even put your name on the front cover and give your books a title (ABC Company, Technology Reference Library), although this is optional. Build your own library of custom books with information you are specifically looking for, while saving countless hours of reading and researching, and arm yourself with C-Level business intelligence.
$99/Quarter or $129/One Time Only (Books arrive within two weeks of each quarter)

B) <u>Access to All Publications by Aspatore</u>

Receive access to hundreds of books and articles already published by Aspatore, or just books and articles in your specialty area, with new publications added every month, to create the ultimate reference library for quick access C-Level business intelligence. Aspatore publishes approximately 60-70 new books every year, in addition to hundreds of articles, briefings, essays and other publications. Our clients use this information to understand the ever-changing needs of their current clients and industries and to learn about current issues facing their potential customer base. Immediately receive access to titles already published (see title list on following pages for titles already published).
i. Electronic Access To Books in Your Specialty Area (Select from: Technology, Legal, Entrepreneurial/Venture Capital, Marketing/Advertising/PR, Management/Consulting) (Via Password Protected Web Site) - $45/Month or $210 for 3 Months Only
ii. Electronic Access to All Books(Via Password Protected Web Site)-$99/Month or $999/Year
iii. Print Publications (All Future Publications by Aspatore, Sent as They are Published)-$1,490 a Year
iv. Print Books-Build Your Own Business Library (65 Best Sellers Already Published by Aspatore) - $1,089 (A savings of 45%)

C) <u>PIA (Personal Intelligence Agent) – Custom Reading Lists</u>

Your quarterly PIA report presents you with information on exactly where to find other business intelligence from newly published books, articles, speeches, journals, magazines, web sites and over 30,000 other business intelligence sources (from every major business publisher in the world) that match your business intelligence profile (the one page questionnaire you fill out describing the type of information you are seeking that is in the business reply envelope). Each 8-10 page report looks like a personalized research report and features sections on the most important new books, articles, and speeches to read, one-sentence descriptions of each, approximate reading times and page counts, and information on the author and publication sources - so you can decide what you should read and how to spend your time most efficiently.
$99 a Year for 4 Reports/Year (Reports arrive within two weeks of start of each quarter.)

To Order, Please Call 1-8<u>66</u>-Aspatore (277-2867) Or Fill in Order Form & Business Intelligence Profile (in Envelope) & Mail or Fax

For Businesses

A) <u>Access to All Publications by Aspatore</u>

Receive print or electronic access to hundreds of books and articles already published by Aspatore, with new publications added every month, creating the ultimate reference library for quick access C-Level business intelligence. This collection will enable you or anyone on your team to get up to speed quickly on a topic, increasing your chances to close more business, identify new areas for business and speak more intelligently with current and prospective clients. Aspatore publishes approximately 40-60 new books every year, in addition to hundreds of articles, briefings, essays and other publications. Simply subscribe to the entire library or books and other publications published only on your area of interest, or make your electronic library available to customers as a resource for them as well.

Titles in Your Industry Only

i. Electronic access to publications in your company's specialty area (Select from: Technology, Legal, Entrepreneurial/Venture Capital, Marketing/Advertising/PR, Management/ Consulting) (Via Password Protected Web Site) - Company employees can access the publications, as often as they like, and printing of the material is permitted. For examples of titles that would be made available immediately, see sample titles page.
Pricing - $999 a month (Based on 1 Yr), $899 a month (Based on 2 Yrs), $799 a month (Based on 5 Yrs), Price includes up to 25 user seats(individuals that can access the web site), Each additional seat is $25 a month

Access to All Titles

ii) Electronic access (Via Password Protected Web Site) to receive every publication published by Aspatore a year. Approximately 60-70 books a year in addition to 50+ books on the sample books page (on the following pages) made available immediately. Anyone in your company can access the publications, as often as they like, and printing of the material is permitted.
Pricing - $1999 a month (Based on 1 Yr), $1899 a month (Based on 2 Yrs), $1799 a month (Based on 5 Yrs), Price includes up to 25 user seats, Each additional seat is $35 a month

Access to All Titles With Additional Navigation

iii) Same as ii, however all publications are arranged by different divisions of your company, each with its own web site, and information can be made available to external customers/clients as well.
Pricing - $2999 a month (Based on 1 Yr), $2899 a month (Based on 2 Yrs), $2799 a month (Based on 5 Yrs), Price includes up to 75 overall user seats and up to 10 different web sites, Each additional seat is $45 a month

iv) Print Publications (All Future Publications by Aspatore, Sent as They are Published)- $1,490 a Year

v) Print Books-Build Your Own Corporate Library (65 Best Sellers Already Published by Aspatore) - $1,089 (A savings of 45%)

To Order, Please Call 1-<u>866</u>-Aspatore (277-2867) Or Fill in Order Form & Business Intelligence Profile (in Envelope) & Mail or Fax

B) <u>Your Own Company Book Every Quarter</u>

Receive 4 quarterly books, each with content from all new books, essays and other publications by Aspatore during the quarter that fits your area of specialty. The content is from over 100 publications (books, essays, journals, briefs) published every quarter on various industries, positions, and topics, available to you months before the general public. Each custom book ranges between 180-280 pages and is based on your company's Business Intelligence Profile. Up to 50 pages of text can be added in each book, enabling you to customize the book for particular practice groups, teams, new hires or even clients. Put your company name on the front cover and give your books a title (ABC Technology, Technology Reference Library), if you like.
Please call 1-866-Aspatore (277-2867) or visit <u>www.Aspatore.com</u> for pricing

C) <u>PIA (Personal Intelligence Agent) – Custom Company Reading Lists</u>

Corporate PIA Reports present your entire company, or a division/group within a company, with information on exactly where to find additional business intelligence from newly published books, articles, speeches, journals, magazines, web sites and over 30,000 other business intelligence sources (from every major business publisher in the world) that match your business intelligence. Each 8-10 page report features sections on the most important new books, articles, and speeches to read, one-sentence descriptions of each, approximate reading times and page counts, and information on the author and publication sources - so you can decide what you should read and how to spend your time most efficiently.
For 1 Report For Entire Company, $499 a Year for 4 Quarterly Reports, Copies Permitted (Reports arrive within two weeks of start of each quarter.)
For Multiple Reports For Same Company, Please call 1-866-Aspatore (277-2867)

D) <u>License Content Published by Aspatore</u>

Our content saves marketing, communications and public relations teams valuable time. For information on licensing content published by Aspatore for a corporate intranet, extranet, newsletter, direct mail, book or in any other way, please email <u>store@aspatore.com</u>.

E) <u>Bulk Orders of Books & Chapter Excerpts</u>

For information on bulk purchases of books or chapter excerpts (specific chapters within a book, bound as their own mini-book), please email <u>store@aspatore.com</u>. For orders over 100 books or chapter excerpts, company logos and additional text can be added to the book. Use for sales and marketing, direct mail and trade show work.

To Order, Please Call 1-<u>866</u>-Aspatore (277-2867) Or Fill in Order Form & Business Intelligence Profile (in Envelope) & Mail or Fax

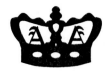

Business Intelligence Profile

Please fill in answers on the page in the envelope or call and answer the questions over the phone.

Your Business Intelligence Profile is Based On:

1. The amount of time you have to spend on reading and analyzing business intelligence every quarter
2. Information you are looking for on your area of specialization and/or industry
3. Your preferred type of business media (books, speeches, magazines, newspapers, Web sites, journals, white papers)
4. Business information most relevant to you (e.g., articles on your industry in a particular periodical)

Sample Questions

Please fill in answers on the page in the envelope or call and answer the questions over the phone.

A: What industries should your PIA report/custom book cover (such as auto, technology, venture capital, real estate, advertising, etc.)?

B: What area of specialty should your PIA report/custom book cover (such as technology, marketing, management, legal, financial, business development)?

C: What level are you at in your career (entry level, manager, VP, CFO, COO, CTO, CMO CEO, etc.) ?

D: What is your preferred source for business intelligence (books, magazines, newspapers, journals, web sites, speeches, interviews)?

E: Are there any particular publications your PIA report should specifically cover (such as The Wall Street Journal, Business Week, books published by Aspatore, etc.)?

F: How many hours do you spend reading business intelligence (books, articles, speeches, interviews) every week? Every month?

G: How many books are you comfortable reading every quarter?

H: Are there any key terms or concepts you are looking to stay on top of (such as nanotechnology, business-to-business marketing, online privacy, etc.)?

I: Is there any other information your PIA should know in order to better customize your quarterly report?

To Order, Please Call 1-866-Aspatore (277-2867) Or Fill in Order Form & Business Intelligence Profile (in Envelope) & Mail or Fax

Praise for Aspatore

"What C-Level executives read to keep their edge and make pivotal business decisions. Timeless classics for indispensable knowledge." - Richard Costello, Manager-Corporate Marketing, General Electric

"True insight from the doers in the industry, as opposed to the critics on the sideline." - Steve Hanson, CEO, On Semiconductor

"Unlike any other business books…captures the essence, the deep-down thinking processes, of people who make things happen." - Martin Cooper, CEO, Arraycomm

"The only useful way to get so many good minds speaking on a complex topic." - Scott Bradner, Senior Technical Consultant, Harvard University

"Easy, insightful reading that can't be found anywhere else." - Domenick Esposito, Vice Chairman, BDO Seidman

"A rare peek behind the curtains and into the minds of the industry's best." - Brandon Baum, Partner, Cooley Godward

"Intensely personal, practical advice from seasoned dealmakers." - Mary Ann Jorgenson, Business Chair, Squire, Sanders & Dempsey

"Become an expert yourself by learning from experts." Jennifer Openshaw, Founder, Women's Financial Network, Inc.

"Real advice from real experts that improves your game immediately." - Dan Woods, CTO, Capital Thinking

"Get real cutting edge industry insight from executives who are on the front lines." - Bob Gemmell, CEO, Digital Wireless

"An unprecedented collection of best practices and insight..." - Mike Toma, CTO, eLabor

"Must have information for business executives." - Alex Wilmerding, Principal, Boston Capital Ventures

"An important read for those who want to gain insight....lifetimes of knowledge and understanding..." - Anthony Russo, Ph.D., CEO, Noonan Russo Communications

"A tremendous treasure trove of knowledge...perfect for the novice or the seasoned veteran."- Thomas Amberg, CEO, Cushman Amberg Comm.

"A wealth of real world experience from the industry leaders you can use in your own business." - Doug Cavit, CTO, McAfee.com

To Order, Please Call 1-866-Aspatore (277-2867) Or Fill in Order Form & Business Intelligence Profile (in Envelope) & Mail or Fax

Sample Books
(Also Available Individually At Your Local Bookstore)

MANAGEMENT/CONSULTING

Empower Profits –The Secrets to Cutting Costs & Making Money in ANY Economy
Building an Empire-The 10 Most Important Concepts to Focus a Business on the Way to Dominating the Business World
Leading CEOs-CEOs Reveal the Secrets to Leadership & Profiting in Any Economy
Leading Consultants - Industry Leaders Share Their Knowledge on the Art of Consulting
Recession Profiteers- How to Profit in a Recession & Wipe Out the Competition
Managing & Profiting in a Down Economy – Leading CEOs Reveal the Secrets to Increased Profits and Success in a Turbulent Economy
Leading Women-What It Takes to Succeed & Have It All in the 21st Century
Management & Leadership-How to Get There, Stay There, and Empower Others
Human Resources & Building a Winning Team-Retaining Employees & Leadership
Become a CEO-The Golden Rules to Rising the Ranks of Leadership
Leading Deal Makers-Leveraging Your Position and the Art of Deal Making
The Art of Deal Making-The Secrets to the Deal Making Process
Management Consulting Brainstormers – Question Blocks & Idea Worksheets

TECHNOLOGY

Leading CTOs-Leading CTOs Reveal the Secrets to the Art, Science & Future of Technology
Software Product Management-Managing Software Development from Idea to Development to Marketing to Sales
The Wireless Industry-Leading CEOs Share Their Knowledge on The Future of the Wireless Revolution
Know What the CTO Knows - The Tricks of the Trade and Ways for Anyone to Understand the Language of the Techies
Web 2.0 – The Future of the Internet and Technology Economy
The Semiconductor Industry-Leading CEOs Share Their Knowledge on the Future of Semiconductors
Techie Talk- The Tricks of the Trade and Ways to Develop, Implement and Capitalize on the Best Technologies in the World
Technology Brainstormers – Question Blocks & Idea Development Worksheets

VENTURE CAPITAL/ENTREPRENEURIAL

Term Sheets & Valuations-A Detailed Look at the Intricacies of Term Sheets & Valuations
Deal Terms- The Finer Points of Deal Structures, Valuations, Term Sheets, Stock Options and Getting Deals Done
Leading Deal Makers-Leveraging Your Position and the Art of Deal Making
The Art of Deal Making-The Secrets to the Deal Making Process
Hunting Venture Capital-Understanding the VC Process and Capturing an Investment
The Golden Rules of Venture Capitalists –Valuing Companies, Identifying Opportunities, Detecting Trends, Term Sheets and Valuations
Entrepreneurial Momentum- Gaining Traction for Businesses of All Sizes to Take the Step to the Next Level
The Entrepreneurial Problem Solver- Entrepreneurial Strategies for Identifying Opportunities in the Marketplace
Entrepreneurial Brainstormers – Question Blocks & Idea Development Worksheets

To Order, Please Call 1-866-Aspatore (277-2867) Or Fill in Order Form & Business Intelligence Profile (in Envelope) & Mail or Fax

LEGAL

Privacy Matters – Leading Privacy Visionaries Share Their Knowledge on How Privacy on the Internet Will Affect Everyone

Leading Lawyers – Legal Visionaries Share Their Knowledge on the Future Legal Issues That Will Shape Our World

Leading Labor Lawyers-Labor Chairs Reveal the Secrets to the Art & Science of Labor Law

Leading Litigators-Litigation Chairs Revel the Secrets to the Art & Science of Litigation

Leading IP Lawyers-IP Chairs Reveal the Secrets to the Art & Science of IP Law

Leading Patent Lawyers –The & Science of Patent Law

Internet Lawyers-Important Answers to Issues For Every Entrepreneur, Lawyer & Anyone With a Web Site

Legal Brainstormers – Question Blocks & Idea Development Worksheets

FINANCIAL

Textbook Finance - The Fundamentals We Should All Know (And Remember) About Finance

Know What the CFO Knows - Leading CFOs Reveal What the Rest of Us Should Know About the Financial Side of Companies

Leading Accountants-The Golden Rules of Accounting & the Future of the Accounting Industry and Profession

Leading Investment Bankers-Leading I-Bankers Reveal the Secrets to the Art & Science of Investment Banking

The Financial Services Industry-The Future of the Financial Services Industry & Professions

MARKETING/ADVERTISING/PR

Leading Marketers-Leading Chief Marketing Officers Reveal the Secrets to Building a Billion Dollar Brand

Emphatic Marketing-Getting the World to Notice and Use Your Company

Leading Advertisers-Advertising CEOs Reveal the Tricks of the Advertising Profession

The Art of PR-Leading PR CEOs Reveal the Secrets to the Public Relations Profession

The Art of Building a Brand –The Secrets to Building Brands

The Golden Rules of Marketing – Leading Marketers Reveal the Secrets to Marketing, Advertising and Building Successful Brands

PR Visionaries-The Golden Rules of PR

Textbook Marketing - The Fundamentals We Should All Know (And Remember) About Marketing

Know What the VP of Marketing Knows –What Everyone Should Know About Marketing, For the Rest of Us Not in Marketing

Marketing Brainstormers – Question Blocks & Idea Development Worksheets

Guerrilla Marketing-The Best of Guerrilla Marketing-Big Marketing Ideas For a Small Budget

The Art of Sales - The Secrets for Anyone to Become a Rainmaker and Why Everyone in a Company Should be a Salesperson

The Art of Customer Service –The Secrets to Lifetime Customers, Clients and Employees Through Impeccable Customer Service

GENERAL INTEREST

ExecRecs- Executive Recommendations For The Best Products, Services & Intelligence Executives Use to Excel

The Business Translator-Business Words, Phrases & Customs in Over 90 Languages

Well Read-The Reference for Must Read Business Books & More...

Business Travel Bible (BTB) – Must Have Information for Business Travelers

Business Grammar, Style & Usage-Rules for Articulate and Polished Business Writing and Speaking

To Order, Please Call 1-866-Aspatore (277-2867) Or Fill in Order Form & Business Intelligence Profile (in Envelope) & Mail or Fax

INSIDE THE MINDS:
THE ART & SCIENCE OF BEING A DOCTOR

Dedications & Acknowledgements

Dr. W. Randolph Chitwood, Jr.

Dedicated to my grandfather, Dr. Edmund Madison Chitwood, and my father, Dr. Walter Randolph Chitwood, Sr., both deceased; acknowledgment to Louise Chut, writer.

Dr. Michael J. Baime

Dedicated to three generations of love and caring: Gloria, Regina, Edwin, and Ian.

Dr. Rosalind Kaplan

I would like to dedicate this chapter to my husband, Dr. Lawrence Kaplan, my true role model and my source of strength.

Dr. Martha S. Grayson, M.D.

I would like to thank my mother, Julie Grayson, my brother, Dr. Paul Grayson, and my friend Dr. Myrtho Montes for their invaluable assistance with the manuscript.

Dr. Nicholas A. DiNubile

I dedicate this to those who helped make me a caring doctor – Connie, Alfred, and Linda – and to those who give me purpose and keep me striving for excellence every day – Emily, Dylan, and Marybeth.

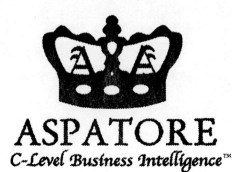

ASPATORE
C-Level Business Intelligence™

Technical mastery
extraordinary musicianship
extreme musicality

deserve a HAYNES